Nail Psoriasis

Dimitris Rigopoulos • Antonella Tosti
Editors

Nail Psoriasis

From A to Z

Springer

Editors
Dimitris Rigopoulos, MD
Department of Dermatology
Athens University School
of Medicine
Athens
Greece

Antonella Tosti, MD
Department of Dermatology
and Cutaneous Surgery
University of Miami
Miller School of Medicine
Miami, FL
USA

ISBN 978-3-319-34573-4 ISBN 978-3-319-08810-5 (eBook)
DOI 10.1007/978-3-319-08810-5
Springer Cham Heidelberg New York Dordrecht London

Printed on acid-free paper

Springer is part of Springer Science+Business Media (www.springer.com)

Preface

Psoriasis is a very common skin condition that clearly influences the quality of life and mental equilibrium of affected patients. Recent research data have expanded greatly our knowledge on psoriasis both in terms of the underlying pathogenetic mechanisms and treatment options. Furthermore, recognition of the fact that the disease does not affect only skin, but is often accompanied with various comorbidities, has changed our point of view on this entity, while new treatment modalities with new therapeutic agents have contributed significantly to the modern view of psoriasis as a systemic disease.

About half of the people who have psoriasis also have changes affecting their nails. Psoriatic nail disease is very variable in appearance and severity. The diversity of clinical appearance in psoriatic nail disease poses exceptional interest to the whole scientific community that is reflected with the huge increase of publications on this topic during the last years.

So, we thought that this is the ideal timing to deal with the state-of-the-art knowledge of nail psoriasis and organize a special book on this topic. In order to cover the full extent of the subject, we invited all those who are considered experts and opinion leaders on this field, to share their knowledge and transfer their valuable experiences on each specific topic of the book.

All medical specialists as dermatologists, rheumatologists, and general practitioners as well as nonmedical professionals as podologists and specialized nurses who deal with psoriatic nail disease in daily practice, will profit from this book. The readers of the book will be able to recognize early signs of the disease, to differentiate them from other nail disorders, to evaluate the severity with validated tools, and to have a comprehensive overview of all modern therapeutic options in order to treat their patients or refer them to the specialist, whenever needed.

Athens, Greece — Dimitris Rigopoulos, MD
Miami, FL, USA — Antonella Tosti, MD

Contents

Contributors

Aurora Alessandrini, MD Department of Specialized, Experimental and Diagnostic Medicine, University of Bologna, Bologna, Italy

Chantel Amarillo, MD Herbert Wertheim College of Medicine, Florida International University, Miami, FL, USA

Zoe Ash, BMedSci, BMBS, MRCP, MD Department of Rheumatology, St. Luke's Hospital, Bradford Teaching Hospitals NHS Foundation Trust, Bradford, UK

Sibel Zehra Aydin, MD Department of Rheumatology, Faculty of Medicine, Koc University, Istanbul, Turkey

Romi Bloom, BS Department of Dermatology and Cutaneous Surgery, University of Miami Leonard M. Miller School of Medicine, Miami, FL, USA

Marie Caucanas, MD Department of Dermatology, Brugmann, St. Pierre and Queen Fabiola Children's University Hospitals, Brussels, Belgium

Carlton Ralph C. Daniel III, MD Clinical Professor of Dermatology, University of Mississippi Medical Center, University of Alabama, Birmingham, AL, USA

Stamatis Gregoriou, MD, PhD Department of Dermatology, University of Athens Medical School, Attikon Hospital, Athens, Greece

Eckart Haneke, MD, PhD Department of Dermatology, Inselspital, Univ Hosp Bern, Bern, Switzerland

Anna Quinn Hare, MD Department of Dermatology, Oregon Health and Science University, Portland, OR, USA

Julie Jefferson, MD Department of Dermatology, Johns Hopkins Medicine, Baltimore, MD, USA

Francisco Kerdel, BSc, MBBS Department of Dermatology, University of Miami Hospital, Miami, FL, USA

Claudia Leon, MD Florida International University College of Medicine, Miami, FL, USA

Dennis McGonagle, PhD, FRCPI Leeds Institute of Rheumatic and Musculoskeletal Medicine and Leeds Musculoskeletal Biomedical Research Unit, Chapel Allerton Hospital, Leeds, UK

Shailee Patel, BS Department of Dermatology and Cutaneous Surgery, University of Miami, Miami, FL, USA

Bianca Maria Piraccini, MD, PhD Dision of Dermatology, Department of Specialized, Experimental and Diagnostic Medicine, University of Bologna, Bologna, Italy

Christos Prevezas, MD Department of Dermatology, Attikon University Hospital, Athens, Greece

Phoebe Rich, MD Department of Dermatology, Oregon Health and Science University, Portland, OR, USA

Bertrand Richert, MD, PhD Department of Dermatology, Brugmann, St. Pierre and Queen Fabiola Children's University Hospitals, Brussels, Belgium

Dimitris Rigopoulos, MD Department of Dermatology, Athens University School of Medicine, Athens, Greece

Rosamary Soto, MD Department of Dermatology, University of Chile, Santiago, RM, Chile

Michela Starace, MD Dision of Dermatology, Department of Specialized, Experimental and Diagnostic Medicine, University of Bologna, Bologna, Italy

Ai Lyn Tan, MRCP, MD Leeds Institute of Rheumatic and Musculoskeletal Medicine and Leeds Musculoskeletal Biomedical Research Unit, Chapel Allerton Hospital, Leeds, UK

Antonella Tosti, MD Department of Dermatology and Cutaneous Surgery, University of Miami Miller School of Medicine, Miami, FL, USA

Ramya Tripuraneni, MBBS Department of Dermatology, University of Miami Hospital, Miami, FL, USA

Ximena Wortsman, MD Department of Radiology and Department of Dermatology, Institute for Diagnostic Imaging and Research of the Skin and Soft Tissue, Clinica Servet, Faculty of Medicine, University of Chile, Santiago, Chile

Natalie C. Yin, BS Department of Dermatology and Cutaneous Surgery, University of Miami, Miami, FL, USA

Martin N. Zaiac, MD Department of Dermatology, Herbert Wertheim College of Medicine, Florida International University, Miami, FL, USA

Greater Miami Skin and Laser Center, Mount Sinai Medical Center, Miami Beach, FL, USA

Epidemiology of Nail Psoriasis 1

Bertrand Richert and Marie Caucanas

Contents

Key Features

- Determining the prevalence of nail psoriasis is utopian.
- There is a positive correlation with the duration and the severity of skin psoriasis.
- Males seem to be more affected.
- Nail psoriasis starts mainly in early adulthood.
- Nail psoriasis carries a high risk of developing psoriatic arthritis.

1.1 Introduction

Physicians often overlook nail psoriasis, and it is difficult to assess its real prevalence. The vast majority of published studies evaluate the prevalence of nail involvement within a study on skin psoriasis. Moreover, several biases are often encountered. This explains why the documented prevalence of nail psoriasis varies between 6.4 and 81.8 %.

B. Richert, MD, PhD (✉) • M. Caucanas, MD
Department of Dermatology, Brugmann, St. Pierre and Queen Fabiola
Children's University Hospitals, Brussels, Belgium
e-mail: bertrand.richert@chu-brugmann.be; marie.caucanas@chu-brugmann.be

D. Rigopoulos, A. Tosti (eds.), *Nail Psoriasis: From A to Z*,
DOI 10.1007/978-3-319-08810-5_1

1.2 History

Using PubMed, Ovid MEDLINE and Ovid EMBASE, a literature search was conducted throughout January 2014, using the keywords nail, psoriasis and epidemiology. Thirty-two articles were selected as they were offering enough data. Among them, 16 were prospective; 11 were retrospective. Five used a questionnaire sent to all patients known as having psoriasis from the data of one or several hospitals [1] or collected from a National Psoriasis Association [2–4] or though a consumer panel [5]. The smallest sample was 44 patients [6] and the largest 11,631 patients [1]. Seven studies focused on children only [7–13].

1.3 Developments

The prevalence of nail psoriasis (NP) has been evaluated through studies on skin psoriasis (see Table 1.1). Some authors evaluated the prevalence of NP in patients hospitalized for exacerbation of skin psoriasis [17] or during the inclusion phase of a clinical trial with a biologic for skin psoriasis [19]. Less than half of the studies are aimed at determining the exact prevalence of specific nail patterns in psoriatic patients [2–4, 7, 14–18, 22, 27, 29, 31]. Very few focus on nail changes as exclusive manifestations of psoriasis in which prevalence varies from 0 to 6 % [8, 14, 23–25]. These patients may not be aware of their disease and may not seek medical advice and, even if they do so, will never be included in a skin psoriasis survey. One study conducted on children showed that in more than half of these children, the nail changes were so subtle that they were not even aware of them [7]. Some patients will only develop a few NP flare-ups over their lifetime and will exhibit completely normal nails the rest of the time. As all published studies performed only a one-time evaluation of the NP, their results do not reflect the real prevalence of NP. This is why some authors deemed it necessary to evaluate the real prevalence of NP over time, by sending a questionnaire to patients, along with pictures of NP, in order to gather information about any past involvement of the nail apparatus [2, 3]. Here there are three main biases: (1) the reliability of patients to diagnose their condition, (2) less than a third of the patients answered the questionnaire and (3) there may be an overestimation of the prevalence of NP, as the questionnaire was sent to members of a patients' association, who were therefore probably more concerned by their disease. Similarly, almost all studies diagnose NP on a clinical basis only and do not even rule out onychomycosis (the main differential diagnosis for NP) with nail clipping, with the exception of a few [7, 14, 17], and a biopsy was only exceptionally carried out [27]. Nail clipping with histological examination looking for the presence of polynuclear neutrophils was never performed. In most studies, the nail involvement is mentioned as a percentage without specifying if the fingers or toenails were affected. In some work, the toenails were not evaluated [16], which is clever, as toenails are not often affected in NP, but nothing looks more like onychomycosis or frictional hyperkeratosis than a hyperkeratotic NP.

Table 1.1 Epidemiologic data from studies dealing with nail psoriasis

Geographical location	Nb	P/R/Q	NPP	A/C	NP M/F ratio	LSPD	LSPS	LPA	1st MCND	2nd MCND	3rd MCND	N/S
Italy [14]	178	P	76.9 %	A	79.8/70.4 %	Yes[a]	Yes	Yes	Onycholysis	Crumbling	SU hyperkeratosis	N
Germany [15]	3,531	P	40.9 %	A	46/34.8 %	Yes	Yes	Yes	/	/	/	N
Spain [16]	661	P	47.4 %	A	53.7/40.2 %	Yes	Yes	Yes	/	/	/	N
France [2]	1,309	QR	60.8 %	A	/	Yes	/	/	SU hyperkeratosis	Whitish aspect	Small spots	N
Poland [17]	106	P	78.3 %	A	/	/	Yes	Yes	SU hyperkeratosis	Pitting	Discoloration	N
The Netherlands [4]	1,728	QR	79.2 %	A+C	/	Yes	/	/	Pitting	Deformation	Onycholysis	N
The Netherlands [3]	1,459	QR	66 %	A	50.8 %/48.2 %	/	/	Yes	Pitting	Onycholysis	Oil-drop	N
Greece [18]	228	P	66.7 %	A	41.4/58.6 %	No	/	No	Oil drop	Onycholysis	Pitting	N
The USA [10]	887	R	17 %	C	/	/	/	/	/	/	/	S
The USA [19]	372	P	81.8 %	A	/	/	No	No	Pitting	Onycholysis	Oil drop	N
Canada [5]	514	Q	26–44 %	A	23/19 %	/	/	Yes	/	/	/	S
Turkey [20]	329	R	16 %	A+C	/	/	/	/	Pitting	SU hyperkeratosis	Onycholysis	S
Turkey [11]	61	R	21.3 %	C	18.2/23.1 %	/	/	/	Pitting	SU hyperkeratosis	Dyschromia	S
Kuwait [13]	190	P	36 %	C	/	/	/	/	Pitting	/	/	S
Kuwait [7]	201	P	37.81 %	C	69.87/39.98 %	No	No	No	Pitting	Onycholysis	SU hyperkeratosis	N
Saudi Arabia [21]	263	R	26.6 %	A	/	/	/	/	/	/	/	S
Nigeria [6]	44	P	15.9 %	A+C	/	/	/	/	/	/	/	S
India [22]	100	P	36 %	A+C	/	/	/	YES	Pitting	SU hyperkeratosis	/	N
India [23]	419	R	31 %	C	/	/	/	/	Pitting	Ridging	Discoloration	S
India [24]	1,000	P	11.5 %	A+C	/	/	/	/	Pitting	SU hyperkeratosis	Thickening	S
India [25]	162	P	74 %	A+C	/	/	/	/	Pitting	Plate thickening	Partial onycholysis	S
Pakistan [26]	515	P	33 %	A+C	/	/	No	No	/	/	/	S
Pakistan [27]	102	P	58 %	A	54/46 %	Yes	Yes	Yes	Roughening	Transverse pitting	Transverse ridging	N
Malaysia [28]	509	R	68 %	A+C	/	/	/	/	/	/	/	S
Malaysia [29]	520	P	65.6 %	A+C	61.3/38.7 %	No	Yes	No	SU hyperkeratosis	Discoloration	Onycholysis	N
Malaysia [30]	138	P	60.9 %	A+C	/	/	/	/	Pitting	Onycholysis	Discoloration	S

(continued)

Table 1.1 (continued)

Geographical location	Nb	P/R/Q	NPP	A/C	NP M/F ratio	LSPD	LSPS	LPA	1st MCND	2nd MCND	3rd MCND	N/S
Singapore [12]	315	R	38 %	C	/	/	/	/	/	/	/	S
Singapore [31]	410	P	78 %	A	1/1	Yes	Yes	Yes	Pitting	Onycholysis	Dystrophy	N
South Korea [32]	5,084	R	26.4 %	A+C	33.5/17.8 %	/	/	/	/	/	/	S
South Korea [33]	4,049	R	27.9 %	A	/	/	/	/	/	/	/	S
China [9]	137	R	25.5 %	C	/	/	/	/	/	/	/	S
Japan [1]	11,631	Q	6.4 %	A+C	66.5/33.5 %	/	/	/	/	/	/	S

Nb number of patients, *P* prospective, *R* retrospective, *Q* questionnaire, *NPP* nail psoriasis prevalence, *A* adults, *C* children, *NP M/F ratio* nail psoriasis male/female ratio, / not applicable, *LSPD* link with skin psoriasis duration, *LSPS* link with skin psoriasis severity, *LPA* link with psoriatic arthritis, *MCND* most common nail dystrophy, *SU* subungual, *N/S* nail or skin study

[a]Not statistically significant but a trend in correlation

The main clinical features of nail psoriasis are often quoted, but the severity of the condition using a scoring (i.e. NaPSI) is not mentioned, except in recent studies [14]. Only two studies report paronychia as a clinical feature of NP [8, 25]. The rate of paronychia was 30 and 2.5 %, respectively. Some recent studies may have collected too much data (body mass index, liver function, lipidogram, PASI, HLA, blood pressure, fasting glucose level, waist circumference, etc.) impairing clear-cut results. Few studies investigated the prevalence of NP in children. In this age group, the prevalence is in a narrower window than studies including adults or adults and children and ranged from 17 to 38 %. The most frequent clinical presentation of NP was pitting, as it is in adults. Only one publication mentions the absence of a link with skin psoriasis severity, the duration of the psoriasis and psoriasis arthropathy. Boys were more commonly affected than girls [7].

Twelve studies included both children and adults [1, 4, 6, 20, 22, 24–26, 28–30, 32] and ten only adults [2, 3, 14–17, 21, 27, 31, 33]. Seven studies found a positive correlation with the severity of skin psoriasis [14–17, 27, 29, 31] and seven with skin psoriasis duration [2, 4, 14–16, 27, 31]. Nine found a correlation with psoriatic arthritis [3, 5, 14–17, 22, 27, 31], with two publications reporting psoriatic arthritis in more than twice as many patients in the NP group as in the unaffected group [15, 16]. Even if several studies mention that NP patients have an early onset of their disease, only two specify the median age of onset [1, 3]. Among the eleven studies reporting the sex ratio of the NP patients, nine found a male predominance, whilst one found an equal ratio [31] and one a female predominance [11]. Very few studies searched for a correlation between familial history of psoriasis and NP: one found that the proportion of patients with a family history of psoriasis was 10.9 % points higher in the nail group compared to the control group [16]. Augustin reported a difference of 11 percentage points higher in men with nail psoriasis compared with men without psoriasis, but the difference was not statistically significant in women [15]. Klaassen found a 64.5 % familial history of psoriasis in the NP patients, but this was not statistically significant ($p=0.153$) [3].

1.4 Outlook: Future Developments

Determining the real prevalence of nail psoriasis over a lifetime seems utopian: the ideal study would be to send a nail expert at regular intervals to a general hospital, for at least one decade, in order to examine the nails of all patients consulting, not only in dermatology but in all departments, and whatever the purpose of consultation. This would give an idea of the prevalence of NP in the general population.

Summary

Few relevant studies of the epidemiology of NP have been published to date. The considerable variation in the prevalence of NP in the literature probably reflects differences in description, definition and methodology used in previous studies. What is highlighted is that NP starts mostly in early adulthood, mostly affects males, is more likely to be associated with severe skin psoriasis and carries a high risk of developing psoriatic arthritis. Pitting is the most common manifestation.

References

1. Takahashi H, Nakamura K, Kaneko F, Nakagawa H, Iizuka H. Analysis of psoriasis patients registered with the Japanese Society for Psoriasis Research from 2002–2008. J Dermatol. 2011;38(12):1125–9.
2. Taieb C, Myon E, Voisard J, Martin N, Corvest M. Nail psoriasis: epidemiological study in France. J Eur Acad Dermatol Venereol. 2005;19(S2):1–411, poster 16–37.
3. Klaassen KMG, van de Kerkhof PCM, Pasch MC. Nail psoriasis: a questionnaire-based survey. Br J Dermatol. 2013;169(2):314–9.
4. de Jong EM, Seegers BA, Gulinck MK, Boezeman JB, van de Kerkhof PC. Psoriasis of the nails associated with disability in a large number of patients: results of a recent interview with 1,728 patients. Dermatology. 1996;193(4):300–3.
5. Papp K, Valenzuela F, Poulin Y, Bernstein G, Wasel N. Epidemiology of moderate-to-severe plaque psoriasis in a Canadian surveyed population. J Cutan Med Surg. 2010;14(4):167–74.
6. Obasi OE. Psoriasis vulgaris in the Guinea Savanah region of Nigeria. Int J Dermatol. 1986;25(3):181–3.
7. Al-Mutairi N, Manchanda Y, Nour-Eldin O. Nail changes in childhood psoriasis: a study from Kuwait. Pediatr Dermatol. 2007;24(1):7–10.
8. Kaur I, Saraswat A, Kumar B. Nail changes in psoriasis: a study of 167 patients. Int J Dermatol. 2001;40(9):601–3.
9. Wu Y, Lin Y, Liu H-J, Huang C-Z, Feng A-P, Li J-W. Childhood psoriasis: a study of 137 cases from central China. World J Pediatr. 2010;6(3):260–4.
10. Tollefson MM, Crowson CS, McEvoy MT, Maradit KH. Incidence of psoriasis in children: a population-based study. J Am Acad Dermatol. 2010;62(6):979–87.
11. Seyhan M, Coşkun BK, Sağlam H, Ozcan H, Karincaoğlu Y. Psoriasis in childhood and adolescence: evaluation of demographic and clinical features. Pediatr Int. 2006;48(6):525–30.
12. Chandran NS, Gao F, Goon ATJ, Chong W, Giam Y, Theng CTS. Clinical characteristics of childhood psoriasis in a multi-ethnic Asian population. J Dermatol. 2012;39(3):278–9.
13. Al-Fouzan AS, Nanda A. A survey of childhood psoriasis in Kuwait. Pediatr Dermatol. 1994;11(2):116–9.
14. Brazzelli V, Carugno A, Alborghetti A, Grasso V, Cananzi R, Fornara L, et al. Prevalence, severity and clinical features of psoriasis in fingernails and toenails in adult patients: Italian experience. J Eur Acad Dermatol Venereol. 2012;26(11):1354–9.
15. Augustin M, Reich K, Blome C, Schäfer I, Laass A, Radtke MA. Nail psoriasis in Germany: epidemiology and burden of disease. Br J Dermatol. 2010;163(3):580–5.
16. Armesto S, Esteve A, Coto-Segura P, Drake M, Galache C, Martínez-Borra J, et al. Nail psoriasis in individuals with psoriasis vulgaris: a study of 661 patients. Actas Dermosifiliogr. 2011; 102(5):365–72.
17. Salomon J, Szepietowski JC, Proniewicz A. Psoriatic nails: a prospective clinical study. J Cutan Med Surg. 2003;7(4):317–21.
18. Kyriakou A, Patsatsi A, Sotiriadis D. Detailed analysis of specific nail psoriasis features and their correlations with clinical parameters: a cross-sectional study. Dermatology. 2011;223(3):222–9.
19. Rich P, Griffiths CEM, Reich K, Nestle FO, Scher RK, Li S, et al. Baseline nail disease in patients with moderate to severe psoriasis and response to treatment with infliximab during 1 year. J Am Acad Dermatol. 2008;58(2):224–31.
20. Kundakci N, Türsen U, Babiker MOA, Gürgey E. The evaluation of the sociodemographic and clinical features of Turkish psoriasis patients. Int J Dermatol. 2002;41(4):220–4.
21. Fatani MI, Abdulghani MH, Al-Afif KA. Psoriasis in the eastern Saudi Arabia. Saudi Med J. 2002;23(2):213–7.
22. Ghosal A, Gangopadhyay, Chanda M, Das N. Study of nail changes in psoriasis. Indian J Dermatol. 2004;49:18–21.
23. Kumar B, Jain R, Sandhu K, Kaur I, Handa S. Epidemiology of childhood psoriasis: a study of 419 patients from northern India. Int J Dermatol. 2004;43(9):654–8.

24. Masood Q, Hassan I, Sameem F, Khan D, Majid I, Singh G, et al. Psoriasis in Kashmir Valley: a clinico-epidemiological study. JK Sci. 2011;13(2):80–3.
25. Bedi TR. Psoriasis in North India. Geographical variations. Dermatologica. 1977;155(5): 310–4.
26. Ejaz A, Raza N, Iftikhar N, Iftikhar A, Farooq M. Presentation of early onset psoriasis in comparison with late onset psoriasis: a clinical study from Pakistan. Indian J Dermatol Venereol Leprol. 2009;75(1):36–40.
27. Ijaz A, Sarwat N. Frequency and pattern of nail changes in patients with nail psoriasis. J Pak Assoc Dermatol. 2009;19:194–9.
28. Chang CC, Gangaram HB, Hussein SH. Malaysian Psoriasis Registry – preliminary report of a pilot study using a newly revised registry form. Med J Malaysia. 2008;63(Suppl C):68–71.
29. Yap FB-B, Pubalan M. Pattern and clinical characteristics of patients with nail psoriasis in Sarawak General Hospital, Malaysia. Indian J Dermatol Venereol Leprol. 2010;76(6):703–4.
30. Yap FB-B. Psoriasis among Sarawakian natives in a tertiary skin centre in Sarawak. Australas J Dermatol. 2010;51(3):210–1.
31. Tham SN, Lim JJ, Tay SH, Chiew YF, Chua TN, Tan E, et al. Clinical observations on nail changes in psoriasis. Ann Acad Med Singapore. 1988;17(4):482–5.
32. Na SJ, Jo SJ, Youn JI. Clinical study on psoriasis patients for past 30 years (1982–2012) in Seoul National University Hospital Psoriasis Clinic. J Dermatol. 2013;40(9):731–5.
33. Kwon HH, Kwon IH, Youn JI. Clinical study of psoriasis occurring over the age of 60 years: is elderly-onset psoriasis a distinct subtype? Int J Dermatol. 2012;51(1):53–8.

Genetics

2

Martin N. Zaiac, Chantel Amarillo, and Claudia Leon

Content

Key Features

- Psoriasis attributes its manifestation to both genetic and environmental factors.
- Consensus has not been established as to the susceptibility allele for psoriasis.
- The genetic foundation responsible for psoriasis variability has proven difficult to decipher.

Psoriasis has been classified as a multifactorial disease. Multifactorial diseases attribute their manifestation to both genetic and environmental factors. The inheritance pattern of psoriasis is not that of a standard single-gene Mendelian pattern of inheritance. Instead, studies have demonstrated that among monozygotic twins,

M.N. Zaiac, MD
Department of Dermatology, Herbert Wertheim College of Medicine, Florida International University, Miami, FL, USA

Greater Miami Skin and Laser Center, Mount Sinai Medical Center, Miami Beach, FL, USA
e-mail: drmartyz@aol.com

C. Amarillo, MD
Herbert Wertheim College of Medicine, Florida International University, Miami, FL, USA

C. Leon, MD
Florida International University College of Medicine, Miami, FL, USA

D. Rigopoulos, A. Tosti (eds.), *Nail Psoriasis: From A to Z*,
DOI 10.1007/978-3-319-08810-5_2

65–70 % concordance exists, and, among dizygotic twins, 15–20 % concordance exists (Farber). If psoriasis was a purely genetically inherited disease, the concordance of monozygotic twins would have approached 100 %. Thus, because the concordance does not show complete penetrance, this is evidence pointing towards other mechanisms of acquiring the disease. Environmental factors include stress, trauma, and infections such as streptococcal pharyngitis [1–3].

Early elucidation of genetic mechanisms relied heavily upon establishing familial patterns of inheritance. A thorough family history was taken, a pedigree chart was formed, and, based on trends of phenotypic expression by individuals, the geneticist would determine if the inheritance was autosomal dominant, autosomal recessive, x-linked, mitochondrial, or another form. Now with the advancement of molecular biology, microsatellite markers can be utilized to determine the pattern of inheritance through their positioning within DNA sequences and identification utilizing specific, commercially developed primers. Microsatellites are sequences of DNA often 1–6 base pairs in length that are repeated within the genome at different locations. These repeats arise from errors in DNA replication called replication slippage, which results in either expansion or contraction in the number of repeats. Often the number of repeats is maintained constant during inheritance between parent and offspring. Primers are used to test individuals within a family demonstrating the phenotype in order to establish putative susceptibility genes and/or alleles in a process known as linkage-based approach. Typically this method is successful for single-gene diseases and less successful for complex diseases such as psoriasis because it involves multiple loci with complex interactions. Another complication is the necessity of a large number of subjects which has been difficult to obtain without an established central database consisting of all individuals phenotypically expressing psoriasis.

Although the linkage-based approach does not contribute much to the determination of pathogenesis of psoriasis, it has provided putative loci for the disease. As technology has improved, better methods have been developed that are capable of comparing two groups: (1) persons with disease and a suspected allele versus (2) those without disease and without the said allele. This method is known as an association study, where microsatellites and single nucleotide polymorphisms (SNPs) are used to analyze a genome within and around a putative susceptibility locus or candidate gene. A SNP is a mutation arising from a substitution, deletion, or insertion of one nucleotide that exists in more than 1 % of the population. From the results, putative loci or genes can then be compared against regions that were proposed via the familial linkage-based approach. The existing setback for such a study is again the number of available subjects with the disease, the involvement of multiple genes, and the financial cost of testing subjects.

Consensus has not been established as to the susceptibility allele for psoriasis. Studies via linkage-based loci have universally confirmed the possibility of the susceptibility allele being present within the locus PSORS1 (a 300-kb region which extends from the HLA-B gene and includes the HLA-C gene) and involving the HLA-C gene located on chromosome 6p21. New developments greatly favor HLA-Cw*0602 as the susceptibility allele at locus PSORS1. This allele suggests that cytotoxic killer T lymphocytes (CD8+ T lymphocytes) are likely to be involved in autoantigen recognition in psoriasis. T cells are thought to recognize epidermal keratin peptides, presented in the context of the Cw6 protein. As psoriasis is a multifactorial disease which involves multiple genes with unpredictable interactions, this complicates understanding the genetic mechanism of inheritance. To date, there are at least 20 genetic loci that have been identified from linkage-based studies. The following is a synopsis of existing literature on the genetics of psoriasis.

Although the susceptibility allele proposed to be located within PSORS1 has been supported by genome-wide linkage and association studies in unstratified trials, when stratifying patients it has been found that several additional loci have suggested involvement. Stratifying patients is a means of adjusting for confounders in epidemiologic studies. Studies stratifying patients according to age of disease onset, site of onset, presence of psoriatic arthritis, and nail involvement led to the strong suggestion of several other PSORS loci in the inheritance of psoriasis.

The PSORS2 locus found on chromosome 17q has been reported, but the location of the risk allele within this locus has been variable from study to study. It may be possible that there is more than one risk allele in this region [4]. PSORS3 was reported on chromosome 4q34, carrying a gene for a protein that regulates the production of *type 1 interferon*. Other studies have shown that type 1 interferon-deficient mice develop psoriasis-like skin lesions. When an association of early-onset psoriasis was seen with this gene, it made it a likely candidate for a susceptibility allele [5]. PSORS9 was reported on 4q31. Several genes reside within this region, and many code for *immunologic proteins*, such as interleukin 15. Antibodies against interleukin 15 have since been successfully tested as treatment on the psoriatic xenografts of mice [6]. PSORS4 resides on chromosome 1q21. It is found within the gene complex involved in *epidermal differentiation*. The genes in this complex encode S100 proteins. S100 proteins are involved in *leukocyte chemotaxis* and are upregulated in the keratinocytes of certain individuals with psoriasis who show linkage to the 1q21 locus [7]. Yet to be confirmed are PSORS5 on chromosome 3q21 and PSOR6 on chromosome 19p13. PSORS6 contains a gene called JUNB [8]. The JUNB is a member of the AP-1 transcription factor family, which controls the *differentiation of keratinocytes*.

The technology of high-volume SNP genotyping has allowed for the creation of extensive catalogs of SNP polymorphisms and LD blocks. As a result, population-based maps of LD haplotypes have been formed. In 2002, the International HapMap Project was launched. The goal of this project is to identify genetic variations between individuals at the population level. By defining subsets of highly informative SNPs ("tag" SNPs), the project aims to identify common patterns. Once more information on tag SNPs becomes available; researchers will then be able to use them in order to locate disease-associated alleles. This curtails the need to use up to ten million SNPs for genome-wide assays and will allow for more efficient genotyping. This approach will likely be used to help identify the remaining susceptibility and disease-modifying alleles in psoriasis.

As mentioned previously, the genetic foundation responsible for psoriasis variability has proven difficult to decipher. Even less is known as to the genetics of nail psoriasis. Many patients with psoriasis experience nail changes, currently estimated at nearly half of all psoriasis patients [9]. More specifically, the subset of patients with psoriatic arthritis have a higher association with experiencing nail changes [10–15]. These nail changes include pitting, "oil drop" spotting, and onychodystrophy. A genetic cause for nail changes has not been verified, yet Julia et al. have identified a variation located at IL1RN that may be responsible for the nail trait in cutaneous psoriasis patients [16]. IL1RN – a regulator of IL-1A proinflammatory activity – has been shown to cause nail changes in children similar to those experienced by psoriasis vulgaris patients [17].

References

1. Gudjonsson JE, Elder JT. Psoriasis. In: Wolff K, Goldsmith LA, Katz SI, Gilchrest BA, Paller AM, Leffell DJ, editors. Fitzpatrick's dermatology in general medicine, vol. 1. New York: McGraw-Hill; 2007. p. 169–94.
2. Lomholt G. Psoriasis: prevalence, spontaneous course, and genetics. In: Published Ph.D Thesis (Lomholt G, ed), Copenhagen: G.E.C. GAC; 1963.
3. Watson W, Cann HM, Farber EM, Nall ML. The genetics of psoriasis. Arch Dermatol. 1972;105:197–207.
4. Samuelsson L, Enlund F, Torinson A, et al. A genome-wide search for genes predisposing to familial psoriasis by using stratification approach. Hum Genet. 1999;105:523–9.
5. Foerster J, Nolte I, Schweiger S, et al. Evaluation of the IRF-2 gene as a candidate for PSORS3. J Invest Dermatol. 2004;122:61–4.
6. Sagoo GS, Tazi-Ahnini R, Barker JW, et al. Meta-analysis of genomewide studies of psoriasis susceptibility reveals linkage to chromosomes 6p21 and 4q28-31. J Invest Dermatol. 2004;122:1401–5.
7. Coto E, Santos-Juanes J, Coto-Segura P, Alvarez V. New psoriasis susceptibility genes: momentum for skin-barrier disruption. J Invest Dermatol. 2011;131(5):1003–5.
8. Zenz R, Eferl R, Kenner L, et al. Psoriasis-like skin disease and arthritis caused by inducible epidermal deletion of Jun proteins. Nature. 2005;437:369–75.
9. Elder JT, Bruce AT, Gudjonsson JE, Johnston A, Stuart PE, Tejasvi T, Voorhees JJ, Abecasis GR, Nair RP. Molecular dissection of psoriasis: integrating genetics and biology. J Invest Dermatol. 2010;130:1213–26.
10. Baker H, Golding DN, Thompson M. The nails in psoriatic arthritis. Br J Dermatol. 1964;76:549–54.
11. Eastmond CJ, Wright V. The nail dystrophy of psoriatic arthritis. Ann Rheum Dis. 1979;38:226–8.
12. Gladman DD, Anhorn KA, Schachter RK, Mervart H. HLA antigens in psoriatic arthritis. J Rheumatol. 1986;13:586–92.
13. Lavaroni G, Kokelj F, Pauluzzi P, Trevisan G. The nails in psoriatic arthritis. Acta Derm Venereol Suppl. 1994;186:113.
14. Williamson L, Dalbeth N, Dockerty JL, Gee BC, Weatherall R, Wordsworth BP. Extended report: nail disease in psoriatic arthritis – clinically important, potentially treatable and often overlooked. Rheumatology. 2004;43:790–4.
15. Wright V. Psoriatic arthritis: a comparative study of rheumatoid arthritis and arthritis associated with psoriasis. Arch Dermatol. 1959;80:27–37.

16. Julia A, Tortosa R, Hernanz JM, Canete JD, Fonseca E, Ferrándiz C, Unamuno P, Puig L, Fernandez-Sueiro JL, Sanmarti R, Rodgriguez J, Gratacos J, Dauden E, Sanchez-Carazo JL, Lopez-Estebaranz JL, Moreno-Ramirez D, Quiero R, Montilla C, Torre-Alonso JC, Perez-Venegas JJ, Vanaclocha F, Herrera E, Munoz-Fernandez S, Gonzalez C, Roig D, Erra A, Acosta I, Fernandez-Nebro A, Zarco P, Alonso A, Lopez-Lasanta M, Garcia-Montero A, Gelpi JL, Absher D, Marsal S. Risk variants for psoriasis vulgaris in a large case-control collection and association with clinical subphenotypes. Hum Mol Genet. 2012;21:4549–57.
17. Aksentijevich I, Masters SL, Ferguson PJ, Dancey P, Frenkel J, van Royen-Kerhoff A, Laxer R, Tedgard U, Cowen EW, Pham TH, et al. An autoinflammatory disease with deficiency of the interleukin-1-receptor antagonist. N Engl J Med. 2009;360:2426–37.

Pathology

3

Eckart Haneke

Contents

Key Features

- Nail psoriasis exhibits most features also seen in psoriasis of the skin, but spongiosis is more often seen in the nail.
- Psoriasis-specific nail lesions are pits and dots, subungual splinter hemorrhages, and leukonychia.
- Acrodermatitis continua suppurativa is a particular form of pustular nail psoriasis.
- Coexistence with onychomycosis is not infrequent.

While some nail changes exhibit histopathologic changes also seen in the skin, others are specific to the nail [1].

Pits are the most common signs of psoriasis [2]. They originate from tiny psoriatic lesions deep in the nail pocket, which are probably analogous to the so-called pinpoint lesions of early psoriasis, i.e., small foci of spongiosis with some lymphocytic exocytosis and very few neutrophils but marked disturbance of the normal keratinization pattern. This translates into circumscribed areas of parakeratosis on the surface of the nail plate as long as this is covered by the ventral

E. Haneke, MD, PhD
Department of Dermatology, Inselspital, Univ Hosp Bern, Bern, Switzerland
e-mail: haneke@gmx.net

D. Rigopoulos, A. Tosti (eds.), *Nail Psoriasis: From A to Z*,
DOI 10.1007/978-3-319-08810-5_3

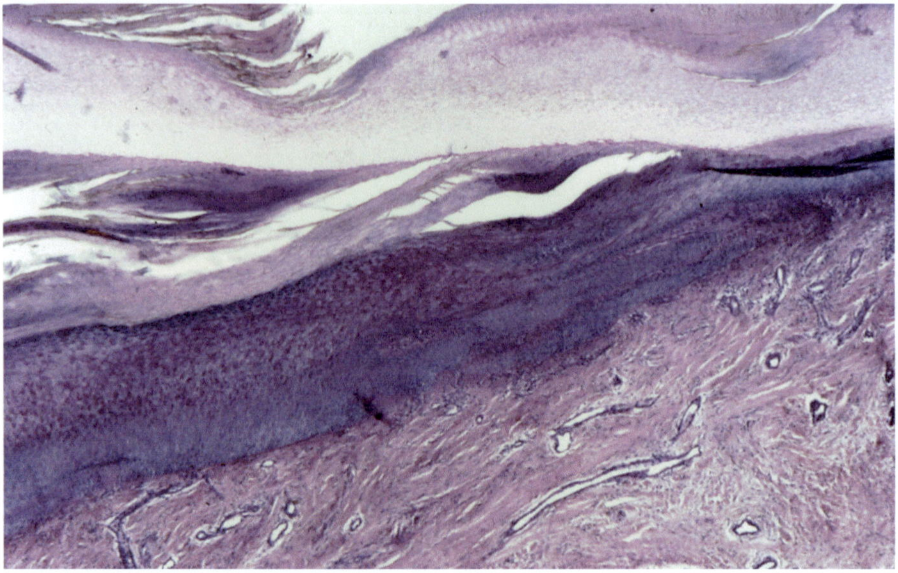

Fig. 3.1 Psoriatic pit with saucer-shaped parakeratosis breaking out of the nail surface as well as parakeratosis with Munro's microabscesses in the subungual keratin

surface of the proximal nail fold. When they grow out, they break off leaving a shallow depression in the nail plate (Fig. 3.1) [3]. However, they may remain stuck to the nail plate and are then clinically seen as small ivory to yellowish dots that are rarely seen beyond the proximal half of the nail. Histopathologically, they are like mounds of parakeratosis [1].

Psoriasis lesions located in the mid-matrix give rise to parakeratosis that is included in the nail plate and clinically seen as a whitish area, called psoriatic leukonychia. Often, they also contain compressed neutrophils. These parakeratosis areas are often arranged in oblique columns from deep proximal to more superficial distal. The matrix epithelium beneath the intraungual parakeratosis is often remarkably unaltered; sometimes mild spongiosis is seen with exocytosis of lymphocytes and neutrophils.

A small acute psoriasis lesion in the matrix is seen as a red spot. Histologically, the matrix demonstrates mild acanthosis, spongiosis, neutrophilic exocytosis, and still relatively little parakeratosis. However, old lesions of the nail matrix and bed psoriasis tend to develop orthokeratosis and a granular layer forming a layered ortho- and parakeratosis [1].

The salmon spot is a lesion analogous to a psoriatic plaque of the skin [2]. The epithelium is often remarkably spongiotic (Fig. 3.2) and acanthotic with long rete ridges and dilated vessels in the papillary dermis reaching high up to the thinned epithelial plate. Minor trauma may cause rupture of the dilated capillaries with erythrocyte accumulation over the papillae that rapidly become included in the subungual keratosis and are seen histopathologically as dense eosinophilic globules, sometimes difficult to

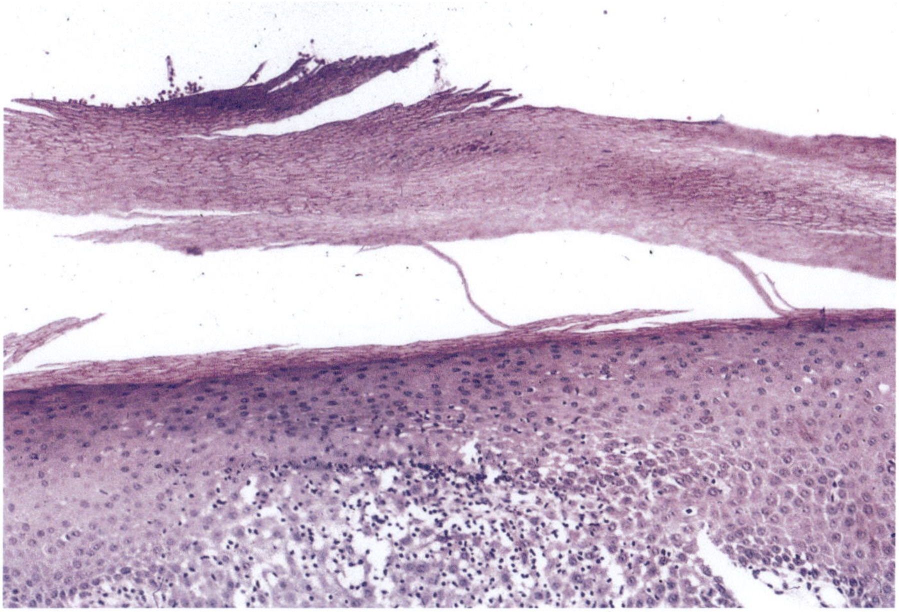

Fig. 3.2 Acute psoriasis of the nail bed with marked spongiosis and lymphocytic exocytosis

distinguish from the eosinophilic subungual keratin. Clinically, they give rise to splinter hemorrhages. In the salmon spot, there is also widespread parakeratosis containing neutrophils forming Munro's microabscesses. These are mainly seen subungually as they start in the nail bed (Fig. 3.1). The subungual keratosis may be enormous with obliquely running columns of parakeratosis with some orthokeratosis (Fig. 3.3) [1].

Psoriasis of the hyponychium and distal nail bed is similar to that of salmon or oil spots. However, the parakeratosis is not firmly attached to the underlying epithelium and tends to break out creating a space under the nail that is macroscopically seen as onycholysis. The histopathology shows an inflammatory infiltrate in the upper dermis with perivascular lymphocytes, long dilated capillaries in the dermal papillae, acanthosis, thinning of the suprapapillary plates, and parakeratosis with various amounts of intermingled neutrophils. Again, old lesions tend to become more orthokeratotic with areas of granular layer [1].

Severe psoriasis of the entire matrix causes nail destruction. There are only remnants of the nail left, often containing neutrophilic microabscesses. The nail plate substance is disorderly arranged with a wavy pattern. Small and large serum inclusions are abundant making the nail intransparent and brittle.

Psoriasis of the proximal nail fold, in particular in patients with psoriatic arthritis, usually causes chronic paronychia-like features with thickening and rounding up of the free margin as well as spontaneous loss of the cuticle. The attachment of the ventral surface of the proximal nail fold with the underlying nail is lost, and the nail plate itself is often thin and contains parakeratotic columns [1]. Again, the common psoriatic features may be seen although they are usually not very pronounced.

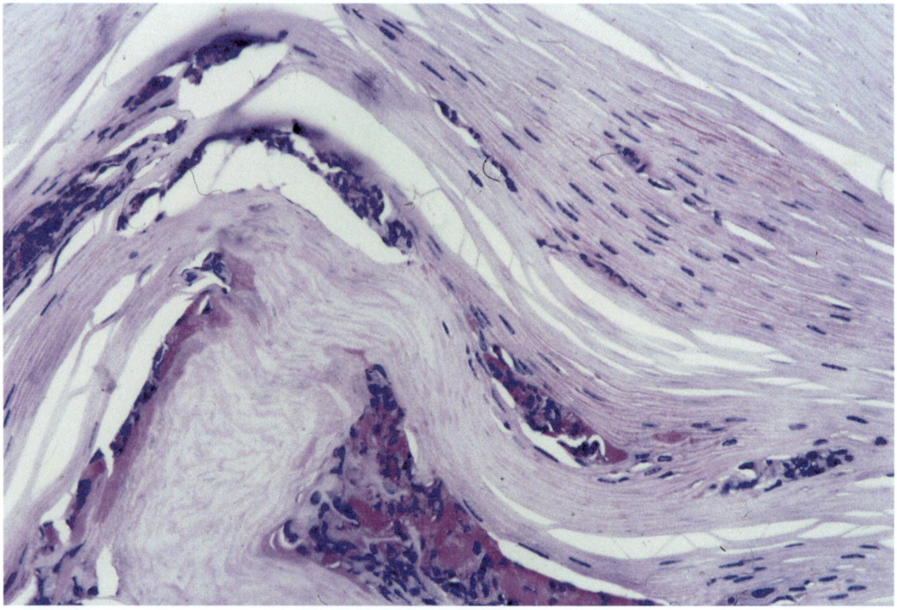

Fig. 3.3 Several Munro's microabscesses in various layers of the subungual hyperkeratosis which is made up of layers of ortho- and parakeratosis. PAS stain

A characteristic feature of psoriasis is the spongiform pustule. This may occur in ordinary nail psoriasis, but above all in the various forms of pustular psoriasis [4]. The matrix and/or nail bed epithelium is thickened, and neutrophils migrate into it accumulating more and more toward the superficial epithelial layers. Finally they form large spongiform pustules with neutrophils lying in a meshwork of keratinocytes that are often very eosinophilic before they become parakeratotic cells; sometimes it is not clear whether this is parakeratinization or more a type of keratinocyte necrosis.

Acrodermatitis continua suppurativa is a particular form of acral pustular psoriasis characterized by the insidious disappearance of the involved nail. Pathologically, all the features of pustular nail psoriasis are exhibited in an exaggerated manner (Fig. 3.4) [1, 4]. There is a tremendous edema of the papillary dermis and exocytosis of huge masses of neutrophils that form spongiform, but sometimes also compact intraepithelial abscesses. The superficial layers of the epithelium become necrotic due to the proteolytic enzymes contained in the masses of neutrophils.

3.1 Differential Diagnosis

A number of different conditions may have to be considered. Pityriasis rubra pilaris often involves the nails with distal subungual hyperkeratosis. Histopathology shows alternating ortho- and parakeratosis, but usually no neutrophilic exocytosis.

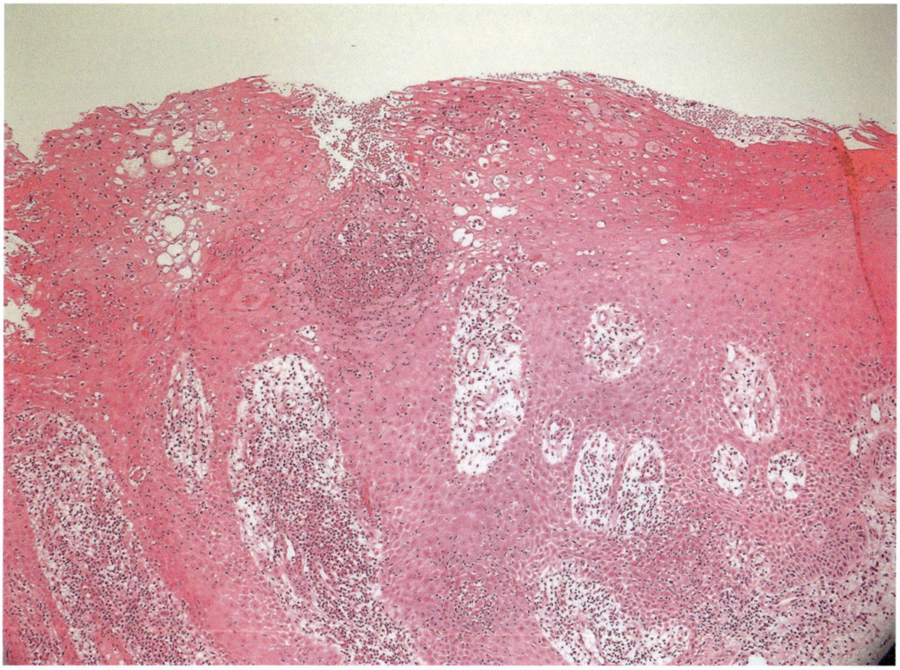

Fig. 3.4 Acrodermatitis continua suppurativa of Hallopeau demonstrates a marked acanthosis, edema of the papillary dermis with dense neutrophilic infiltrate containing some eosinophils, and neutrophilic exocytosis with spongiform pustule formation

In Sézary's syndrome, there may be subungual hyperkeratosis containing pyknotic lymphocytes difficult to distinguish from intracorneal leukocytes. The most important differential diagnosis is onychomycosis. Depending on the type of onychomycosis and the severity, a marked subungual hyperkeratosis may develop often containing Munro's microabscesses. A PAS stain is therefore essential in all cases of suspected nail psoriasis and onychomycosis. However, the amount of parakeratosis is less in fungal nail infections, not arranged in oblique columns, and pits are not or only very rarely seen. Fungal hyphae and spores are easily identified with special stains (Table 3.1). It has to be stressed, however, that serum inclusions are PAS positive due to their content of glycoproteins and that they may be small and fusiform mimicking fungal elements. In contrast to them, serum is homogeneously positive, whereas fungal elements have their cell walls demonstrated. The problem is further compounded by the fact that both conditions can coexist in the same nail (Fig. 3.5). Reiter's syndrome of the nail is almost identical to pustular psoriasis, but there are more extravasated erythrocytes. Simple onycholysis may mimic nail psoriasis. Onycholysis semilunaris is due to overzealous manicure. The normal papillomatous pattern of the undersurface of the nail plate is smooth because it is scratched off. Eczema also affects the nail. It essentially presents a spongiotic dermatitis with large areas of spongiosis of both the matrix and nail bed with spongiotic vesicle

Table 3.1 Histopathologic differential diagnosis of psoriasis and onychomycosis

	Psoriasis	Onychomycosis
Subungual hyperkeratosis	Marked subungual hyperkeratosis with accumulation of neutrophils and serum globules	Marked subungual hyperkeratosis with accumulation of neutrophils and serum globules
Nail bed and matrix granulosis	Focal hypergranulosis	Focal hypergranulosis
Nagelbett hyperplasia	Papillomatous nail bed hyperplasia	Papillomatous nail bed hyperplasia
Spongiosis and exocytosis	Spongiosis, mononuclear and neutrophilic exocytosis	Spongiosis and mononuclear exocytosis
Surface alterations	Pitlike surface depressions with parakeratosis or parakeratotic mounds	Rarely present
Demonstration of fungi	Usually not seen, but possible in coexistent onychomycosis	Hyphae and spores in the subungual hyperkeratosis and ventral nail plate

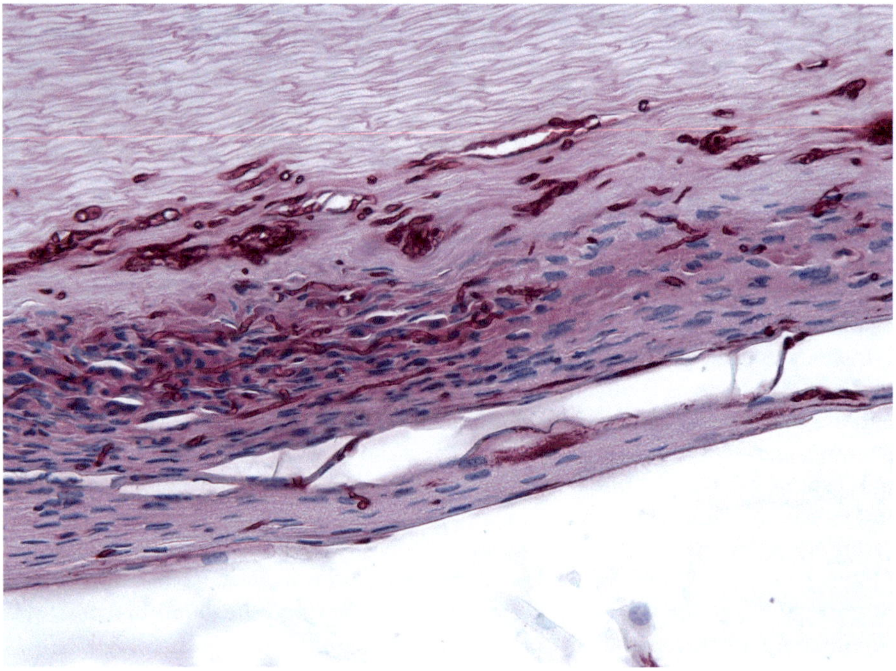

Fig. 3.5 Coexistence of severe psoriasis and onychomycosis. The patient had been treated for widespread psoriasis with nail involvement with a biologic, all the nails except the one shown here cleared. Histology shows Munro's microabscess and masses of fungal elements with relatively large caliber. PAS stain

formation, but without neutrophilic exocytosis. Toxic contact dermatitis may be indistinguishable [5]. Hypertrophic lichen planus may cause a mixed pattern of lichenoid and eczematous changes. Alopecia areata is also a spongiotic dermatitis that, however, only affects the matrix and rarely develops spongiotic vesicles, and these are smaller than in eczema. Serum globules in the nail plate may be abundant giving the nail a thickened and intransparent aspect.

References

1. Haneke E. Nail psoriasis. In: Soung J, Koo B, editors. Psoriasis. Rijeka: Intech; 2011. ISBN 978-953-307-878.
2. Zaias N. Psoriasis of the nail: a clinical-pathologic study. Arch Dermatol. 1969;99:567–79.
3. Jiaravuthisan MM, Sasseville D, Vender RB, Murphy F, Muhn CY. Psoriasis of the nail: anatomy, pathology, clinical presentation, and a review of the literature on therapy. J Am Acad Dermatol. 2007;57:1–27.
4. Piraccini BM, Fanti PA, Morelli R, Tosti A. Hallopeau's acrodermatitis continua of the nail apparatus: a clinical and pathological study of 20 patients. Acta Derm Venereol. 1994;74:65–7.
5. Takeuchi S, Matsuzaki Y, Ikenaga S, Nishikawa Y, Kimura K, Nakano H, Sawamura D. Garlic-induced irritant contact dermatitis mimicking nail psoriasis. J Dermatol. 2011;38:280–2.

Comorbidities of Nail Psoriasis: From A to Z

4

Ramya Tripuraneni and Francisco Kerdel

Contents

Key Features

- Psoriasis is a multisystem chronic inflammatory disorder with numerous associated comorbidities.
- HLA B27 is positive in 50 % of cases of spondyloarthritis, and it is significant to note that psoriatic arthritis is affiliated with a higher risk of developing nail involvement than is plaque psoriasis alone.

R. Tripuraneni, MBBS (✉) • F. Kerdel, BSc, MBBS
Department of Dermatology, University of Miami Hospital, Miami, FL, USA
e-mail: ramya.tripuraneni@gmail.com; dr.kerdel@fadcenter.com

D. Rigopoulos, A. Tosti (eds.), *Nail Psoriasis: From A to Z*,
DOI 10.1007/978-3-319-08810-5_4

- TNF-alpha, which is a major inflammatory mediator in psoriasis, has a predominant role in the induction of insulin resistance. Insulin resistance in turn causes endothelial dysfunction, which creates an atherogenic environment that may lead to vascular inflammation, atherosclerosis, thrombosis, and ultimately a myocardial infarction or stroke.
- Psoriasis is linked with an increased risk of lymphoproliferative malignancies with the greatest association being between psoriasis and cutaneous T cell lymphoma (CTCL). It is postulated that the abnormal immunogenic response in psoriasis leads to an elevated risk of lymphoma due the increased B and T cell activity.
- Regular monitoring and screening for comorbidities should be carried out which includes blood pressure monitoring, lipid panel, CBC, serum glucose levels, and renal function tests to screen for cardiometabolic disease, renal disease, as well as malignancies.

4.1 Introduction

Nail psoriasis is a common and disabling manifestation of cutaneous plaque-type psoriasis that affects the patient both functionally and psychologically. The prevalence of nail involvement in psoriatic patients ranges from 7 to 56 %, with the lifetime incidence being as high as 80–90 % [1]. Nail psoriasis is a frequent ailment among patients and a great source of disability. Nail manifestations can be associated with pain, an altered sense of touch, and a functional impairment in dexterity resulting in an inability to grab small objects. All these conditions culminate in a restriction of daily activities, psychological stress, low self-esteem, and a reduced quality of life [2].

Psoriasis, being an inflammatory skin disease, has a wide array of systemic effects and associated comorbidities. Some of the common encountered comorbidities associated with psoriasis are cardiometabolic dysfunction and psoriatic arthritis. Diabetes, metabolic syndrome, and depression are also frequently encountered. Patients with moderate to severe psoriasis have a greater probability of developing comorbid conditions than those who have a mild form of the disease. Severe psoriasis has additionally been linked with a 3.5–4.4 reduction in life expectancy when compared to the general population. It is imperative that dermatologists be well versed with the associated extracutaneous manifestations of psoriasis, as well as the debilitating effects of nail psoriasis, so that they may be able to effectively prevent, counsel, and treat their patients.

4.2 Epidemiology

Psoriasis occurs worldwide and has no gender predilection. In the USA, psoriasis affects nearly 2 % of the general population, which roughly corresponds to 7.5 million people. Psoriasis is less common in specific ethnic groups, such as Africans,

Japanese, Eskimos, Australians, and Norwegians [3, 4]. Psoriasis can present at any age; however, a bimodal age of onset is characteristic. The majority of cases, approximately 75 %, present before the age of 40 years. Patients with early disease onset usually have a positive family history of psoriasis, frequent association with HLA-Cw6, and a more severe disease.

4.3 History

Historically, psoriasis was believed to be exclusively a skin disease, but over the years researchers have found many links to internal manifestations. In the 1980s, the immune system was postulated to be the primary pathogenesis of psoriasis. It is currently believed that this abnormal immunogenic response of psoriasis is a common underlying entity linking psoriasis to its numerous comorbidities.

4.4 Clinical Features

Psoriasis is typically associated with the presence of inflammatory plaques on the skin. As mentioned earlier, there has been increasing evidence that recognizes psoriasis as being a multisystemic chronic inflammatory disorder with numerous associated comorbidities. Examples of extracutaneous disorders that have been linked to psoriasis include psoriatic arthritis, obesity, metabolic syndrome, type II diabetes, and cardiovascular, cerebrovascular, and peripheral vascular diseases [5]. Other associated comorbidities include malignancy such as lymphoma, nonalcoholic fatty liver disease, chronic kidney disease, and inflammatory bowel disease. Furthermore, these patients may suffer from psychiatric disorders such as depression and more frequently smoke and abuse alcohol. All these conditions can cause serious morbidity and be associated with an increased mortality [6].

It is conceived that the unifying link between these diseases is a common pathogenicity. Psoriasis and its recognized comorbidities are chronic proinflammatory disorders powered by a similar expression of immune response mechanisms. In psoriatic lesions, as well as the peripheral blood, there are elevated levels of T helper (TH) cells, mainly TH1 and TH17. Elevated levels of the TH1 cytokine, IFN-γ, and the TH17 cytokines, IL-17A and IL-22, which are responsible for the local and systemic inflammation, also accompany these cells. Further causative factors include a shared genetic susceptibility, adverse response of prescribed medications, and environmental factors such as smoking and alcohol use.

4.4.1 Psoriatic Arthritis

Psoriatic arthritis is the most common comorbidity associated with psoriasis. It is thought that it may be part of the natural progression of the same disease and not necessarily a comorbidity. If left untreated it can lead to destruction of the joint and have a negative impact on the patient's quality of life (Fig. 4.1). HLA B27 is positive in

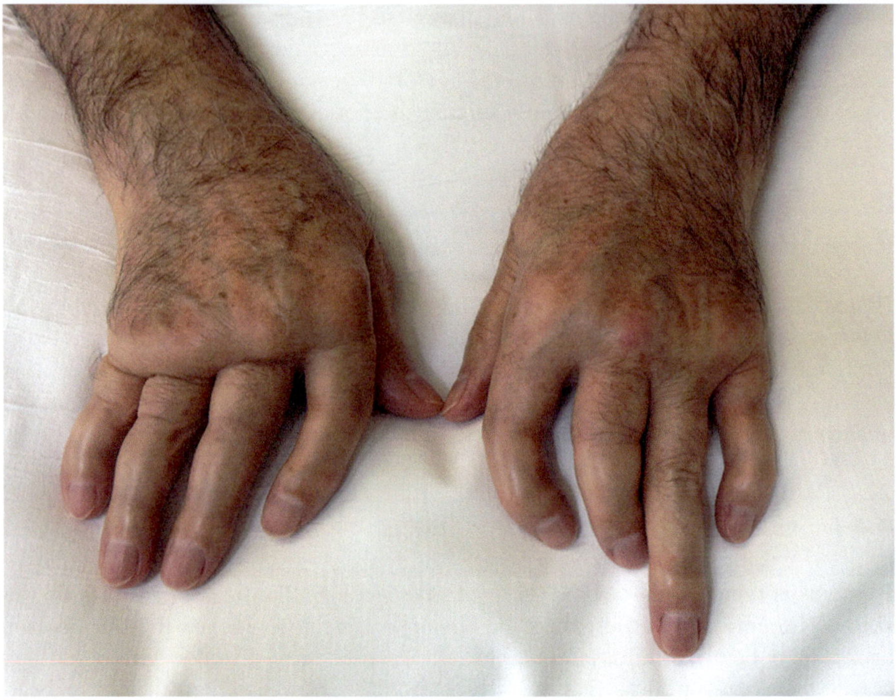

Fig. 4.1 Psoriatic arthritis (arthritis mutilans)

50 % of cases of spondyloarthritis, and it is significant to note that psoriatic arthritis is affiliated with a higher risk of developing nail involvement than is plaque psoriasis alone. It is speculated that this is secondary to inflammation of the enthesis around the DIP, which is thought to be a continuation of the supporting fascia of the nail [7–9]. The different types of psoriatic arthritis are outlined in Table 4.1. Clinical manifestations of nail involvement are dependent on the anatomic part of the nail that is affected. If psoriasis involves the nail matrix, it can present as pitting, ridging, leukonychia, or crumbling. If psoriasis involves the nail bed, it may present as discoloration (salmon patches and oil drops/spots), splinter hemorrhages, subungual hyperkeratosis or onycholysis [10, 11]. In addition to the above symptoms of psoriasis of nails, patients may also have an associated fungal infection of the nail in addition to nail psoriasis. Fungal infections if left untreated can worsen the nail psoriasis.

4.4.2 Cardiometabolic Dysfunction

The theory of the "psoriatic march" proposes that systemic inflammation in severe psoriasis can cause insulin resistance [12]. TNF-alpha, which is a major inflammatory mediator in psoriasis, has a predominant role in the induction of insulin

Table 4.1 Types of psoriatic arthritis

Symmetric arthritis
Affects the same joints on both sides of the body
Asymmetric arthritis
Affects any joint, such as the wrist, hip, knee, etc.
Affected joints are warm, tender, red, and enlarged
Enlarged "sausage digits" can occur when fingers and toes are involved
Distal interphalangeal predominant (DIP)
Commonly confused with osteoarthritis
Affects DIP of fingers and toes
Commonly associated with nail psoriasis
Spondylitis
Inflammation of the spinal column
May present with stiffness involving the neck, lower back, or pelvic girdle
Arthritis mutilans
Affects less than 5 % of psoriatic arthritis patients
Severe, deforming, and destructive form of arthritis
Predominantly affects the small joints of the hands and feet

Table 4.2 Components of metabolic syndrome

Hypertriglyceridemia (>150 mg/dL)
Low HDL (men <40 mg/dL, women <50 mg/dL)
Insulin resistance (fasting glucose >100 mg/dL)
Abdominal obesity (waist circumference in men >40 in., women >35 in.)
Hypertension (blood pressure >140/90 mmHg)

resistance. Insulin resistance in turn causes endothelial dysfunction, which creates an atherogenic environment that may lead to vascular inflammation, atherosclerosis, thrombosis, and ultimately a myocardial infarction or stroke. This is the underlying cause of cardiovascular, cerebrovascular, peripheral vascular disease, hypertension, as well as type II diabetes mellitus [12, 13]. It is also thought that psoriatic patients have a higher prevalence of cardiovascular risk factors, such as obesity and smoking when compared with individuals without psoriasis.

Metabolic syndrome is a combination of medical disorders that, when occurring simultaneously, increases an individual's chance of developing diabetes and cardiovascular disease. Constituents of metabolic syndrome are outlined in Table 4.2. Insulin resistance and abdominal obesity are underlying risk factors for metabolic syndrome. Additionally, elevated levels of proinflammatory factors such as TNF-alpha, IL-6, and C-reactive protein are also associated with the development of metabolic syndrome [14]. It has been theorized that fat cells also play a role as inflammatory mediators by releasing adipocytokines, hormones, and free fatty acids [15]. Recent studies have concluded that psoriasis patients have a higher propensity to develop metabolic syndrome as well as the individual components of metabolic syndrome [16]. In an investigational study done to detect the prevalence of metabolic syndrome in psoriatic patients, Love et al. concluded that the prevalence of metabolic syndrome was an estimated 40 % in psoriatics and 23 % in the control group (patients without psoriasis). The study consisted of 6,549 participants that nationally represented men and women between the ages of 20 and 59 years [17]. In obese patients, weight loss has been linked with a reduction in the serum concentrations of inflammatory mediators, such as TNF-alpha, IL-6, C-reactive protein, and fibrinogen. There is also a simultaneous increase in adiponectin, which exhibits anti-inflammatory and insulin-sensitizing properties [18].

4.4.3 Gastrointestinal Disease

Nonalcoholic fatty liver disease (NAFLD) is a clinical spectrum that extends from benign fatty liver disease to steatohepatitis and may ultimately result in liver cirrhosis or hepatocellular carcinoma. It has been postulated that psoriasis, NAFLD, and metabolic syndrome are strongly interconnected. NAFLD is thought to be a consequence of obesity and insulin resistance and is therefore considered to be the hepatic manifestation of metabolic syndrome. There are several theories that support the relationship between psoriasis and NAFLD. One theory proposes that visceral adipocytes release free fatty acids, adipocytokines, and hormones that result in inflammation. Another theory suggests that proinflammatory cytokines induce insulin resistance and patients with psoriasis with the maximum resistance develop NAFLD.

Inflammatory bowel disease (IBD), which includes Crohn's disease and ulcerative colitis, is a chronic inflammatory state. Patients with IBD develop psoriasis at a higher rate than the general population. It is also believed that the incidence of IBD in psoriasis is seven times higher than the general population [19]. Psoriasis and IBD share a common immunogenic pathway, which is reflective in the efficacy of medications that block TNF-alpha for the treatment of both diseases. Furthermore, Crohn's disease and psoriasis share genetic susceptibility loci, which are localized to chromosome 6p21 locus in the MHC region. Another shared gene among the two diseases is the gene that encodes the IL-23 receptor and IL-12B.21. In the serum and skin of psoriatics and the lamina propria of Crohn's disease, there are elevated levels of IL-17 and IL-23 [20]. Crohn's disease is much more common in psoriasis patients than in ulcerative colitis. Even though the association between UC and psoriasis is not as common, it is still statistically significant.

4.4.4 Chronic Kidney Disease

It has been established that there is an association between patients with moderate to severe psoriasis and chronic kidney disease (CKD). Psoriasis is an independent risk factor for developing CKD and end stage renal disease. Patients with psoriasis and patients with CKD have abnormalities in gut flora. The belief is that the alteration in the gut flora alters the intestinal lining, thereby allowing excessive toxic material to be absorbed. The relative risk of developing chronic kidney disease is highest among younger patients with severe psoriasis. This has warranted CKD screening in psoriasis.

4.4.5 Lymphoma

Psoriasis is linked with an increased risk of lymphoproliferative malignancies. The greatest association is between psoriasis and cutaneous T cell lymphoma (CTCL), followed by Hodgkin's lymphoma. It is postulated that the abnormal immunogenic response in psoriasis leads to an elevated risk of lymphoma due the increased B and T cell activity. The upregulated immune response that occurs in psoriatic patients causes an increased number of circulating B and T lymphocytes that can eventually result in a lymphoproliferative malignancy. Additionally, treatment with immunosuppressive medications used in psoriasis may be an independent risk factor, or it may be that having psoriasis and being exposed to immunomodulating medications can result in an increased chance of developing lymphomas. It is important to consider this elevated risk of CTCL when trying to therapeutically managing these patients. The immunosuppressive properties of biologics, which are frequently used in severe psoriasis, can increase the incidence of lymphoma development [21].

4.4.6 Psychological Disease

The psychological burden of psoriasis can be substantial, and patients with more severe psoriasis tend to bear a greater psychological strain. Many patients with moderate to severe psoriasis suffer from depression, depressive symptoms, and suicidal ideation. Psoriasis has been linked to a decrease in the quality of life, difficulty performing daily activities, and the onset of depression. Patients with psoriasis are known to suffer from physical, emotional, and psychosocial stressors, which leads to a higher prevalence of depression and anxiety. There is evidence that suggests the increased levels of TNF-alpha and IL-1 in psoriasis may be linked to chronic fatigue and depression and that TNF blockade has lead to clinical improvement as well as improved affect [22]. It has been shown that psoriatic patients perceive their disease to negatively impact their quality of life to a level comparable to patients suffering from a chronic illness such as cancer, heart disease, and major depression [2]. It has also been documented that patients with severe psoriasis have been linked to higher rates of alcohol consumption. This is thought to be related to the negative impact the disease has on the individual's quality of life, leading to depression and consequently heavy alcohol use. Reducing these stressors through active therapeutic disease control and utilizing methods of stress reduction can be of great benefit to these patients.

4.5 Diagnostic Clues

Once a patient has an established diagnosis of psoriasis, regular monitoring and screening for comorbidities should be carried out. This entails blood work including a lipid panel, CBC, serum glucose levels, and renal function tests to screen for cardiometabolic disease, renal disease, as well as malignancies. Joint evaluation should be carried out to check for joint swelling, erythema, and obvious deformities. Specifically, patients who have nail involvement should be evaluated for psoriatic arthritis since there is a higher incidence of this when nail psoriasis is present. Patients should also have their blood pressure checked at each visit and should be questioned on their mental and emotional state to exclude psychological disease. Inquiries should be made into the lifestyle of patient in order to identify modifiable habits such as diet, smoking, and alcohol consumption.

Summary

Psoriasis is a chronic, multifactorial disorder, which encompasses the interaction of a multitude of genetic and environmental risk factors. In addition to affecting the skin, psoriasis is associated with physical and emotional comorbidities, which have a negative bearing on the quality of life of the affected patients. It is important for the dermatologist to be well versed with the associated comorbidities of psoriasis. This allows for early detection of the various comorbidities and thus reducing preventable morbidity and mortality.

References

1. de Berker DAR, Baran R, Dawber RPR. The nail in dermatological diseases. In: Baran R, Dawber RPR, de Berker DAR, Haneke E, Tosti A, editors. Baran and Dawber's diseases of the nails and their management. 3rd ed. Malden: Blackwell Science; 2001. p. 172–222.
2. Gulliver W. Long-term prognosis in patients with psoriasis. Br J Dermatol. 2008;159 Suppl 2:2–9.
3. Raychaudhuri SP, Farber EM. The prevalence of psoriasis in the new world. J Eur Acad Dermatol Venereol. 2001;15:16–7.
4. Christophers E. Psoriasis- epidemiology and clinical spectrum. Clin Exp Dermatol. 2001;26: 314–20.
5. Onumah N, Kircik L. Psoriasis and its comorbidities. J Drugs Dermatol. 2012;11 Suppl 5: s5–10.
6. Abuabara K, Azfar RS, Shin DB, et al. Cause-specific mortality in patients with severe psoriasis: a population-based cohort study in the United Kingdom. Br J Dermatol. 2010; 163:586–92.
7. Williamson L, Dalbeth N, Dockerty JL, Gee BC, Weatherall R, Wordsworth BP. Extended report: nail disease in psoriatic arthritis – clinically important, potentially treatable and often overlooked. Rheumatology (Oxford). 2004;43(6):790–4.
8. Tan AL, Benjamin M, Toumi H, et al. The relationship between the extensor tendon enthesis and the nail in distal interphalangeal joint disease in psoriatic arthritis – a high resolution MRI and histological study. Rheumatology (Oxford). 2007;46(2):253–6.
9. McGonagle D. Enthesitis: an autoinflammatory lesion linking nail and joint involvement in psoriatic disease. J Eur Acad Dermatol Venereol. 2009;23 Suppl 1:9–13.
10. Jiaravuthisan MM, Sasseville D, Vender RD, Murphy F, Muhn CY. Psoriasis of the nail: anatomy, pathology, clinical presentation, and a review of the literature on therapy. J Am Acad Dermatol. 2003;49(2):206–12.
11. Reich K. Approach to managing patients with nail psoriasis. J Eur Acad Dermatol Venereol. 2009;23 Suppl 1:15–21.
12. Boehncke WH, Boehncke S, Tobin AM, Kirby B. The 'psoriatic march' a concept of how severe psoriasis may drive cardiovascular comorbidity. Exp Dermatol. 2011;20:303–7.

13. Boehncke WH, Boehncke S. Research in practice: the systemic aspects of psoriasis. J Dtsch Dermatol Ges. 2008;6(8):622–5.
14. Gottlieb A, Chao C, Dann F. Psoriasis comorbidities. J Dermatolog Treat. 2008;19:5–21.
15. Gisondi P, Del Giglo M, Cozzi A, Girolomino G. Psoriasis, the liver, and the gastrointestinal tract. Dermatol Ther. 2010;23:155–9.
16. Vena GA, Vestita M, Cassano N. Can early treatment with biologics modify the natural history of comorbidities? Dermatol Ther. 2010;23(2):181–93.
17. Love TJ, Qureshi AA, Karlson EW, Gelfand JM, Choi HK. Prevalence of the metabolic syndrome in psoriasis: results from the National Health and Nutrition Examination Survey, 2003–2006. Arch Dermatol. 2011;147(4):419–24.
18. Madsen EL, Rissansen A, Brunn JM. Weight loss larger than 10 % is needed for general improvement of levels of circulating adiponectin and markers of inflammation in obese subjects: a 3 year weight loss study. Eur J Endocrinol. 2008;158(2):179–87.
19. Di Cesare A, Di Meglio P, Nestly FO. The Il-23/Th17 axis in the immunopathogenesis of psoriasis. J Invest Dermatol. 2009;129:1339–50.
20. Wolf N, Quaranta M, Prescott NJ, et al. Psoriasis is associated with pleiotropic susceptibility loci identified in type II diabetes ad Crohn disease. J Med Genet. 2008;45:114–6.
21. Gelfand JM, Shin D, et al. The risk of lymphoma in patients with psoriasis. J Invest Dermatol. 2006;126:2194–201.
22. Patarca R, Kimas NG, Lugtendorf S, Antoni M, Fletcher MA. Dysregulated expression of tumor necrosis factor in chronic fatigue syndrome: interrelations with cellular sources and patterns of soluble immune mediator expression. Clin Infect Dis. 1994;18 Suppl 1:147S–53.

Arthritis

5

Zoe Ash, Sibel Zehra Aydin, Ai Lyn Tan,
and Dennis McGonagle

Contents

Key Features

- Psoriatic arthritis occurs in approximately 20 % of people with psoriasis.
- Psoriatic nail disease is more common amongst those with PsA than those with skin psoriasis alone.
- Nail disease in psoriasis is a predictor of PsA development.
- Nail disease in psoriasis is associated with subclinical remote enthesopathy.

Z. Ash, BMedSci, BMBS, MRCP, MD
Department of Rheumatology, St. Luke's Hospital, Bradford Teaching Hospitals NHS Foundation Trust, Bradford, UK
e-mail: zoe.ash@bthft.nhs.uk

S.Z. Aydin, MD
Department of Rheumatology, Faculty of Medicine, Koc University, Istanbul, Turkey
e-mail: drsibelaydin@gmail.com

A.L. Tan, MRCP, MD • D. McGonagle, PhD, FRCPI (✉)
Leeds Institute of Rheumatic and Musculoskeletal Medicine and Leeds Musculoskeletal Biomedical Research Unit, Chapel Allerton Hospital, Leeds, UK
e-mail: a.l.tan@leeds.ac.uk; d.g.mcgonagle@leeds.ac.uk

D. Rigopoulos, A. Tosti (eds.), *Nail Psoriasis: From A to Z*,
DOI 10.1007/978-3-319-08810-5_5

- Imaging studies in PsA have shown a strong association between nail disease and bony involvement of the distal phalanx or inflammation at the extensor tendon insertion.
- Treatments used for PsA may also improve the psoriatic nail disease.

5.1 Introduction

Psoriatic arthritis (PsA) is a subtype of the spondyloarthritides (SpA) and occurs in association with psoriasis. It has been known since the 1950s that people with PsA are more likely to have nail disease than those with skin psoriasis alone. Furthermore, the presence of nail disease in a patient with psoriasis appears to be a harbinger for the future development of PsA. Imaging studies have led to a greater understanding of the pathogenesis of the nail abnormalities, but how this can be applied clinically is still not well defined. The relationship is less clear between psoriasis and nail disease in subjects without clinical arthritis. Treatments that work for PsA generally also help the nail disease. The purpose of this chapter is to discuss the link between nail disease and PsA.

5.2 Epidemiology

Psoriatic arthritis occurs in 0.1 % of the general population with an equal sex distribution, and a peak incidence in the fifth decade [1]. Studies assessing the prevalence of PsA amongst psoriasis patients have shown varying figures, largely due to the methodology and the populations studied. Overall it is thought to occur in approximately 20 % of people with psoriasis [2, 3]. The duration of psoriasis is associated with an increased risk of developing PsA [3]. In the majority of cases, the onset of skin disease occurs first, with arthritis developing a number of years later [4]. Occasionally a simultaneous onset occurs which has been historically noted in cases with nail psoriasis [5]. A small proportion of people with PsA do not develop skin psoriasis at all, but in most of these cases there is a family history of psoriasis. Occasionally the only visible cutaneous manifestation of PsA may be nail disease. Estimates of the prevalence of PsA in different populations worldwide vary significantly, with a very low prevalence reported in Japan and a much higher prevalence in Europe and North America [6]. This may relate to study methodology but also variations in the prevalence of psoriasis as well as genetic and environmental factors.

5.3 History

An association between psoriasis and arthritis was first reported as early as 1818 and was further described in a series of publications by Moll and Wright from the 1950s and later [5, 7–9]. Another key discovery was the ability to distinguish PsA from rheumatoid arthritis (RA) by the use of the rheumatoid factor blood test which was noted to be negative in the PsA groups [10]. The recognition that enthesitis (as determined by MRI and ultrasound imaging) was common in PsA leads to an appreciation of the importance of this lesion as a unifying concept. This leads to anatomical studies and imaging studies of psoriatic nails showing a link with enthesopathy and a unifying concept for the whole spectrum of joint and nail disease.

5.4 Clinical Features

Psoriatic arthritis may present with pain, swelling or stiffness of the affected joints. Stiffness which is worse in the morning, lasting for at least 30 min, is typical of an inflammatory arthritis. These symptoms may be episodic with complete resolution at times or may be continuously progressive. Associated systemic features include malaise, fatigue and anaemia of chronic disease, the latter of which is much less common now due to earlier disease presentations. Blood tests may also show raised inflammatory markers including ESR and CRP, but these are more likely to be normal in PsA in comparison to RA. PsA is a heterogenous disease with multiple possible manifestations. These include inflammation of the peripheral joints, inflammation at the entheses (tendon or ligament insertions), dactylitis (swelling of a whole digit) and involvement of the axial skeleton. A number of typical patterns of peripheral joint disease have been described [9], including predominant distal interphalangeal (DIP) joint involvement, arthritis mutilans (a highly destructive arthritis with bone lysis and telescoping of the digits), a symmetrical polyarthritis similar to RA, an asymmetrical oligoarthritis and predominant axial disease similar to ankylosing spondylitis. Patients may evolve from one pattern to another and may have features of more than one type. There is also a wide variation in the severity of the disease, from patients who experience one self-limiting episode of a monoarthritis to those with a progressive destructive arthritis which causes joint deformity, disability and pain. There can be considerable difficulty distinguishing between PsA and differential diagnoses such as osteoarthritis even amongst expert rheumatologists. Thus the treatment is tailored depending on the severity of both the arthritis and psoriasis in a particular patient. Untreated, PsA may cause bone damage visible on radiographs which leads to functional impairment. There is good evidence that all of the newer biologic treatments available prevent progression of this damage [11].

5.5 Diagnostic Clues

The diagnosis of PsA is a clinical one made by a rheumatologist, based on a typical history and examination findings. The rheumatoid factor is usually negative, but a positive rheumatoid factor does not exclude the diagnosis in the presence of features characteristic for PsA. Radiographs of the hands and feet may be helpful, both to detect typical features of PsA and to exclude other diagnoses.

Table 5.1 Moll and Wright criteria

The presence of psoriasis
An inflammatory arthritis (peripheral arthritis and/or sacroiliitis or spondylitis)
The (usual) absence of serological tests for rheumatoid factor

Table 5.2 The CASPAR criteria

Inflammatory articular disease (joint, spine or entheseal) (*mandatory*)	
Plus, 3 or more points from the following:	
Evidence of current psoriasis, a personal history of psoriasis or a family history of psoriasis	
Current psoriasis is defined as psoriatic skin or scalp disease present today as judged by a rheumatologist or dermatologist	Score 2
A personal history of psoriasis is defined as a history of psoriasis that may be obtained from a patient, family physician, dermatologist, rheumatologist, or other qualified health care providers	Score 1
A family history of psoriasis is defined as a history of psoriasis in a first- or second-degree relative according to the patient report	Score 1
Typical psoriatic nail dystrophy including onycholysis, pitting and hyperkeratosis observed on current physical examination	Score 1
A negative test for the presence of rheumatoid factor by any method except latex but preferably by enzyme-linked immunosorbent assay or nephelometry, according to the local laboratory reference range	Score 1
Either current dactylitis, defined as swelling of an entire digit, or a history of dactylitis recorded by a rheumatologist	Score 1
Radiographic evidence of juxta-articular new bone formation, appearing as ill-defined ossification near joint margins (but excluding osteophyte formation) on plain radiographs of the hand or foot	Score 1

Historically, the Moll and Wright criteria (Table 5.1) were used to classify patients for research studies, but these have been largely superseded by the CASPAR criteria (Table 5.2) [12]. These are not diagnostic criteria but are intended to help select homogenous populations of patients for study. The CASPAR criteria have the advantage that they do allow the inclusion of patients without skin psoriasis, in the presence of sufficient other typical features.

The differential diagnoses of PsA include RA, osteoarthritis and gout, all of which can occur in patients with psoriasis. A careful history and examination along with blood tests (to assess for RA and gout) and radiographs are necessary to enable a firm diagnosis.

Studies have found that a significant proportion of psoriasis patients have undiagnosed PsA [13, 14]. A number of simple screening tools have been developed to aid dermatologists, primary care physicians and others involved in their care to identify those patients who would benefit from a rheumatology assessment. These include the Psoriasis Epidemiology Screening Tool (PEST) [15], the Toronto Psoriatic Arthritis Screen (ToPAS) [16], the Psoriatic Arthritis Screening and Evaluation (PASE) tool [17], the Psoriatic and Arthritic Questionnaire (PAQ) [18] and the Early ARthritis for Psoriatic patients (EARP) [19].

5.6 Nail Disease and Psoriatic Arthritis

Increasing evidence supports that nail disease and arthritis are not just frequent findings related to psoriasis but they are also linked to each other. From the clinical point of view, nail disease is more common in PsA patients than psoriasis patients [20]. Nail psoriasis is also more prevalent in patients with severe psoriasis, those aged over 50 and those with a longer duration of psoriasis [21]. It is most frequently seen in the dominant thumb nail, suggesting a possible role of trauma or "Koebnerisation" in its development [22]. Observational studies have shown that the presence of nail disease in a psoriasis patient is a predictor for the later development of PsA, as is the presence of scalp psoriasis or intergluteal psoriasis [23]. In PsA, there is a well-recognised association between nail disease and DIP joint arthritis [24–29].

The pathogenesis of nail disease in PsA has been studied using a variety of imaging techniques. Radiographs are a simple cheap way to study the bones but do not assess the soft tissues such as the tendons and the nails, nor do they allow detection of inflammation in or around the joint. Radiographs are however useful for assessing bony damage and in the diagnosis.

Magnetic resonance imaging (MRI) has found increasing use in a research setting for examining the nail, DIP joint and surrounding structures. Using MRI, inflammation in the soft tissues as well as the bone can be seen (Fig. 5.1). Features

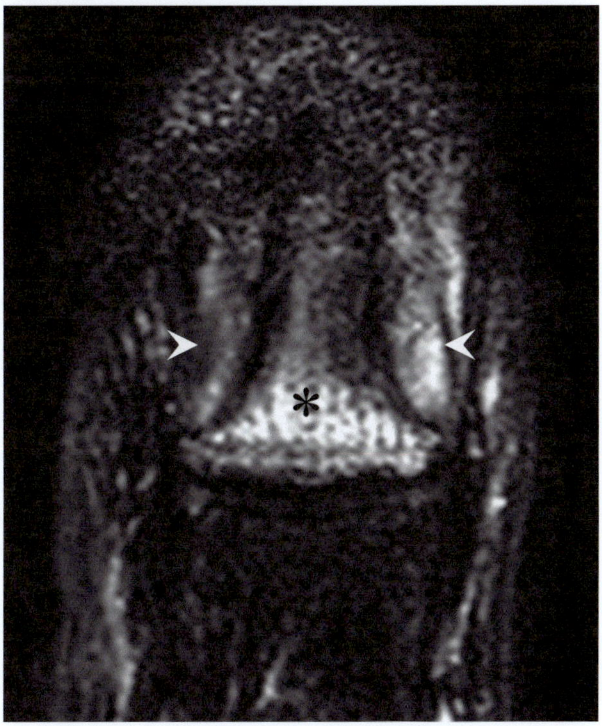

Fig. 5.1 T2 fat-suppressed coronal MRI of a distal interphalangeal joint of a 17-year-old female with PsA. There is diffuse high signal affecting the distal phalange (*asterisk*) and the nail bed (*arrow heads*)

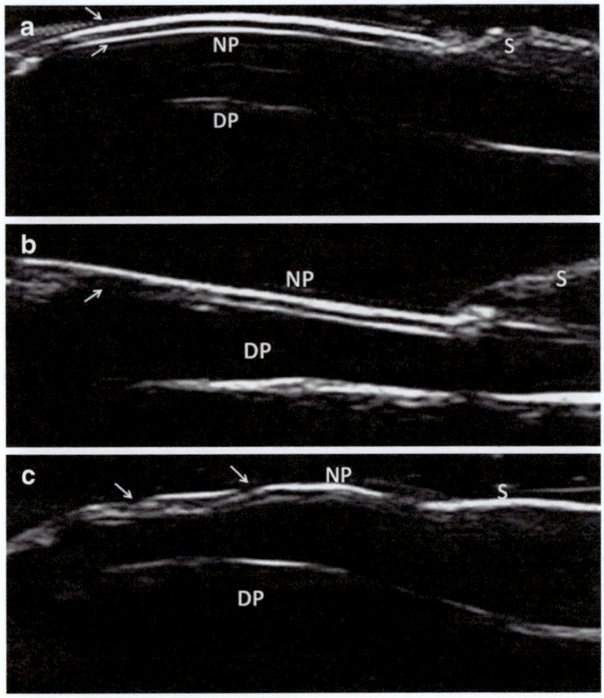

Fig. 5.2 (**a**) Longitudinal scan of the healthy nail demonstrating the trilaminar structure as two hyperechoic lines (*arrows*) surrounding an anechoic line. (**b**) Loss of the trilaminar appearance at the ventral plate seen as the irregularity and absence of the deeper hyperechoic line (*arrow*). (**c**) Pitting and irregularity of the nail plate (*arrows*). *NP* nail plate, *S* skin, *DP* distal phalanx, *DIPJ* DIP joint

of bony damage such as erosions are detected at an earlier stage than with radiographs. In a cross-sectional study using MRI scans, active arthritis of the DIP joint in PsA was found to represent diffuse inflammation not just of the joint but also of the entheses, ligaments, bone and other extracapsular structures [30]. This inflammation extended up to the nail bed. This was further studied using cadaveric histology, and here it was seen that the nail matrix is very closely associated with fibres from the extensor tendon enthesis in particular, but also the flexor tendon and collateral ligaments [31]. These are all entheseal structures which are commonly involved in DIP joint PsA, and this led to the hypothesis that inflammation at the entheses disturbs the normal process of nail formation, leading to the presence of nail disease.

Magnetic resonance imaging studies have also shown that clinical nail disease is visible as thickening of the nail, and that PsA patients with nail disease universally have bony involvement of the distal phalanx and are more likely to have DIP arthritis than those with clinically normal nails [32]. A small observational study showed a link between bone oedema on a baseline MRI scan and the later development of onycholysis and hyperkeratosis [33].

Ultrasound has been used to study the nail in PsA. The nail has a typical trilaminar appearance in health. In patients with PsA and nail disease, thickening of the nail plate and bed is seen, with loss of the trilaminar appearance [34, 35] (Fig. 5.2). In a cohort of patients with psoriatic nail disease, a good correlation was seen between the ultrasound appearances of the nail and the clinical modified NAPSI

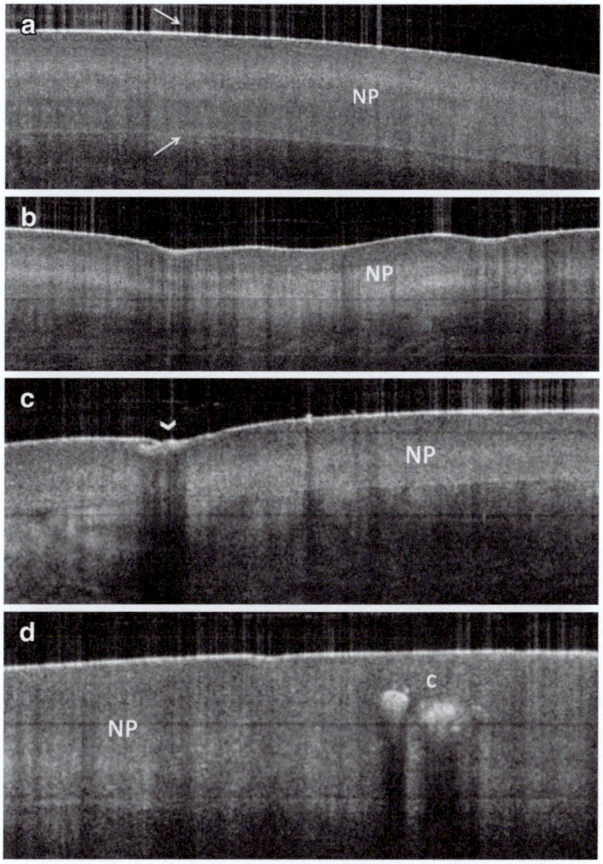

Fig. 5.3 (**a**) The typical appearance of the healthy nail by OCT. The superficial and the deeper layers of the nail plate (*NP*) are clearly marked (*arrows*). (**b**) Irregularity of the superficial nail plate in a patient with psoriatic nail disease seen as waving of the superficial layer. (**c**) Focal pitting (*arrow head*) with an underlying shadow. (**d**) Calcifications within the nail plate seen as hyperreflective spots (*c*) with an underlying shadow

score for nail disease [36]. Other than the ability of ultrasound to visualise the nail, studies have also investigated the link between nail disease and enthesitis using ultrasound. In a recent study, an association was seen between extensor tendon thickening and nail disease in both PsA and psoriasis patients [36]. In addition, another study showed that there is an increased risk of subclinical enthesitis detected by ultrasound in psoriasis patients if they have nail disease, thus supporting the systemic nature of the inflammation [37]. Curiously, there was also a relationship seen between the severity of the nail disease as measured by the modified NAPSI and the degree of subclinical enthesopathy.

Recently, optical coherence tomography (OCT) has been used to study the nail. This gives extremely high-resolution images of the nail plate and allows more accurate measurement of the nail thickness, despite limitations of being unable to image the deeper tissues like the matrix or the adjacent enthesis [38]. The characteristic appearances of a number of psoriatic nail disease manifestations have now been described, and the meaning of each individual lesion awaits for further validation [39] (Fig. 5.3). Thus far, nail disease in PsA and nail disease in psoriasis cases have similar appearances.

Advances in imaging have given greater resolution and higher sensitivity to detect structural changes and inflammation of very superficial tissues such as the nail. The more we understand about the disease pathogenesis in psoriasis, the better chance there will be to predict the risk of developing arthritis at follow-up.

Summary for the Clinician

Psoriatic arthritis is a common form of arthritis in psoriasis patients. Awareness of PsA amongst clinicians caring for patients with psoriasis in primary and secondary care may allow for an earlier diagnosis to be made. This facilitates the choice of a treatment that will improve both the skin and the joints but also prevent the joint damage that occurs in untreated PsA. The clinician should be aware that the presence of nail psoriasis is a pointer to a regional and systemic subclinical enthesopathy like picture and confers a higher risk of the development of PsA.

References

1. Shbeeb M, Uramoto KM, Gibson LE, O'Fallon WM, Gabriel SE. The epidemiology of psoriatic arthritis in Olmsted County, Minnesota, USA, 1982–1991. J Rheumatol. 2000;27(5):1247–50.
2. Zachariae H. Prevalence of joint disease in patients with psoriasis: implications for therapy. Am J Clin Dermatol. 2003;4(7):441–7.
3. Gelfand JM, Weinstein R, Porter SB, Neimann AL, Berlin JA, Margolis DJ. Prevalence and treatment of psoriasis in the United Kingdom: a population-based study. Arch Dermatol. 2005;141(12):1537–41.
4. Gladman DD, Shuckett R, Russell ML, Thorne JC, Schachter RK. Psoriatic arthritis (PSA) – an analysis of 220 patients. Q J Med. 1987;62(238):127–41.
5. Wright V. Psoriasis and arthritis. Ann Rheum Dis. 1956;15(4):348–56.
6. Alamanos Y, Voulgari PV, Drosos AA. Incidence and prevalence of psoriatic arthritis: a systematic review. J Rheumatol. 2008;35(7):1354–8.
7. Alibert JLM. Précis théorique et pratique sur les maladies de la peau. Paris: Caille et Ravier; 1818.
8. Wright V. Psoriatic arthritis. A comparative radiographic study of rheumatoid arthritis and arthritis associated with psoriasis. Ann Rheum Dis. 1961;20:123–32.
9. Moll JM, Wright V. Psoriatic arthritis. Semin Arthritis Rheum. 1973;3(1):55–78.
10. Blumberg BS, Bunim JJ, Calkins E, Pirani CL, Zvaifler NJ. ARA nomenclature and classification of arthritis and rheumatism (tentative). Arthritis Rheum. 1964;7:93–7.
11. Ash Z, Gaujoux-Viala C, Gossec L, Hensor EM, FitzGerald O, Winthrop K, et al. A systematic literature review of drug therapies for the treatment of psoriatic arthritis: current evidence and meta-analysis informing the EULAR recommendations for the management of psoriatic arthritis. Ann Rheum Dis. 2012;71(3):319–26.
12. Taylor W, Gladman D, Helliwell P, Marchesoni A, Mease P, Mielants H. Classification criteria for psoriatic arthritis: development of new criteria from a large international study. Arthritis Rheum. 2006;54(8):2665–73.
13. Khraishi M, Chouela E, Bejar M, Landells I, Hewhook T, Rampakakis E, et al. High prevalence of psoriatic arthritis in a cohort of patients with psoriasis seen in a dermatology practice. J Cutan Med Surg. 2012;16(2):122–7.
14. Haroon M, Kirby B, FitzGerald O. High prevalence of psoriatic arthritis in patients with severe psoriasis with suboptimal performance of screening questionnaires. Ann Rheum Dis. 2013;72(5):736–40.
15. Ibrahim GH, Buch MH, Lawson C, Waxman R, Helliwell PS. Evaluation of an existing screening tool for psoriatic arthritis in people with psoriasis and the development of a new

instrument: the Psoriasis Epidemiology Screening Tool (PEST) questionnaire. Clin Exp Rheumatol. 2009;27(3):469–74.
16. Gladman DD, Schentag CT, Tom BD, Chandran V, Brockbank J, Rosen C, et al. Development and initial validation of a screening questionnaire for psoriatic arthritis: the Toronto Psoriatic Arthritis Screen (ToPAS). Ann Rheum Dis. 2009;68(4):497–501.
17. Husni ME, Meyer KH, Cohen DS, Mody E, Qureshi AA. The PASE questionnaire: pilot-testing a psoriatic arthritis screening and evaluation tool. J Am Acad Dermatol. 2007;57(4):581–7.
18. Alenius GM, Stenberg B, Stenlund H, Lundblad M, Dahlqvist SR. Inflammatory joint manifestations are prevalent in psoriasis: prevalence study of joint and axial involvement in psoriatic patients, and evaluation of a psoriatic and arthritic questionnaire. J Rheumatol. 2002;29(12):2577–82.
19. Tinazzi I, Adami S, Zanolin EM, Caimmi C, Confente S, Girolomoni G, et al. The early psoriatic arthritis screening questionnaire: a simple and fast method for the identification of arthritis in patients with psoriasis. Rheumatology (Oxford). 2012;51(11):2058–63.
20. Brazzelli V, Carugno A, Alborghetti A, Grasso V, Cananzi R, Fornara L, et al. Prevalence, severity and clinical features of psoriasis in fingernails and toenails in adult patients: Italian experience. J Eur Acad Dermatol Venereol. 2012;26(11):1354–9.
21. Tham SN, Lim JJ, Tay SH, Chiew YF, Chua TN, Tan E, et al. Clinical observations on nail changes in psoriasis. Ann Acad Med Singapore. 1988;17(4):482–5.
22. Rich P, Griffiths CE, Reich K, Nestle FO, Scher RK, Li S, et al. Baseline nail disease in patients with moderate to severe psoriasis and response to treatment with infliximab during 1 year. J Am Acad Dermatol. 2008;58(2):224–31.
23. Wilson FC, Icen M, Crowson CS, McEvoy MT, Gabriel SE, Kremers HM. Incidence and clinical predictors of psoriatic arthritis in patients with psoriasis: a population-based study. Arthritis Rheum. 2009;61(2):233–9.
24. Green FA. Distal interphalangeal joint disease and nail abnormalities. Ann Rheum Dis. 1968; 27(1):55–9.
25. Jones SM, Armas JB, Cohen MG, Lovell CR, Evison G, McHugh NJ. Psoriatic arthritis: outcome of disease subsets and relationship of joint disease to nail and skin disease. Br J Rheumatol. 1994;33(9):834–9.
26. Cohen MR, Reda DJ, Clegg DO. Baseline relationships between psoriasis and psoriatic arthritis: analysis of 221 patients with active psoriatic arthritis. Department of Veterans Affairs Cooperative Study Group on Seronegative Spondyloarthropathies. J Rheumatol. 1999;26(8):1752–6.
27. Kane D, Stafford L, Bresnihan B, FitzGerald O. A classification study of clinical subsets in an inception cohort of early psoriatic peripheral arthritis – 'DIP or not DIP revisited'. Rheumatology (Oxford). 2003;42(12):1469–76.
28. Scarpa R, Manguso F, Oriente A, Peluso R, Atteno M, Oriente P. Is the involvement of the distal interphalangeal joint in psoriatic patients related to nail psoriasis? Clin Rheumatol. 2004;23(1):27–30.
29. Williamson L, Dalbeth N, Dockerty JL, Gee BC, Weatherall R, Wordsworth BP. Extended report: nail disease in psoriatic arthritis – clinically important, potentially treatable and often overlooked. Rheumatology (Oxford). 2004;43(6):790–4.
30. Tan AL, Grainger AJ, Tanner SF, Emery P, McGonagle D. A high-resolution magnetic resonance imaging study of distal interphalangeal joint arthropathy in psoriatic arthritis and osteoarthritis: are they the same? Arthritis Rheum. 2006;54(4):1328–33.
31. Tan AL, Benjamin M, Toumi H, Grainger AJ, Tanner SF, Emery P, et al. The relationship between the extensor tendon enthesis and the nail in distal interphalangeal joint disease in psoriatic arthritis – a high-resolution MRI and histological study. Rheumatology (Oxford). 2007;46(2):253–6.
32. Scarpa R, Soscia E, Peluso R, Atteno M, Manguso F, Del Puente A, et al. Nail and distal interphalangeal joint in psoriatic arthritis. J Rheumatol. 2006;33(7):1315–9.
33. Dalbeth N, Pui K, Lobo M, Doyle A, Jones PB, Taylor WJ, et al. Nail disease in psoriatic arthritis: distal phalangeal bone edema detected by magnetic resonance imaging predicts development of onycholysis and hyperkeratosis. J Rheumatol. 2012;39(4):841–3.
34. Gisondi P, Idolazzi L, Girolomoni G. Ultrasonography reveals nail thickening in patients with chronic plaque psoriasis. Arch Dermatol Res. 2012;304(9):727–32.

35. Gutierrez M, Filippucci E, De Angelis R, Filosa G, Kane D, Grassi W. A sonographic spectrum of psoriatic arthritis: "the five targets". Clin Rheumatol. 2010;29(2):133–42.
36. Aydin SZ, Castillo-Gallego C, Ash ZR, Marzo-Ortega H, Emery P, Wakefield RJ, et al. Ultrasonographic assessment of nail in psoriatic disease shows a link between onychopathy and distal interphalangeal joint extensor tendon enthesopathy. Dermatology. 2012;225(3):231–5.
37. Aydin SZ, Ash ZR, Tinazzi I, Castillo-Gallego C, Kwok C, Wilson C, et al. The link between enthesitis and arthritis in psoriatic arthritis: a switch to a vascular phenotype at insertions may play a role in arthritis development. Ann Rheum Dis. 2013;72(6):992–5.
38. Sattler E, Kaestle R, Rothmund G, Welzel J. Confocal laser scanning microscopy, optical coherence tomography and transonychial water loss for in vivo investigation of nails. Br J Dermatol. 2012;166(4):740–6.
39. Aydin SZ, Castillo-Gallego C, Ash ZR, Abignano G, Marzo-Ortega H, Wittmann M, et al. Potential use of optical coherence tomography and high-frequency ultrasound for the assessment of nail disease in psoriasis and psoriatic arthritis. Dermatology. 2013;227(1):45–51.

The Clinical Features of Nail Psoriasis

6

Romi Bloom and Antonella Tosti

Contents

Key Features

- Pitting and onycholysis are the most common clinical manifestations of nail psoriasis.
- The frequency of clinical features differs in the fingernails versus toenails.
- Nail matrix changes include nail pitting, leukonychia, red spots in the lunula, and crumbling.
- Nail bed abnormalities include onycholysis, splinter hemorrhages, hyperkeratosis, and "oil-drop" salmon patch discoloration.
- The quality of life in patients with nail psoriasis is lower than in psoriasis patients without nail involvement.

R. Bloom, BS
Department of Dermatology and Cutaneous Surgery,
University of Miami Leonard M. Miller School of Medicine, Miami, FL, USA
e-mail: rbloom1@med.miami.edu

A. Tosti, MD (✉)
Department of Dermatology and Cutaneous Surgery, University of Miami
Miller School of Medicine, Miami, FL, USA
e-mail: antonella.tosti@unibo.it

D. Rigopoulos, A. Tosti (eds.), *Nail Psoriasis: From A to Z*,
DOI 10.1007/978-3-319-08810-5_6

6.1 Introduction

Nail involvement is present in over half of patients with psoriasis and consequently has a prominently negative impact on society [1, 2]. The clinical gamut of nail involvement is diverse and includes changes to the nail matrix, the nail bed, or both [3]. The main nail matrix dystrophy is nail pitting while onycholysis, subungual hyperkeratosis, splinter hemorrhages, and oil-drop discoloration are the major nail bed findings [4]. Lesions of the nail plate are due to the location of disease in the nail matrix as well as the duration of the disease [5]. This chapter will describe the broad array of clinical features of nail psoriasis in order to help clinicians identify the condition, which will enable dermatologists to treat the symptoms and hopefully improve patients' lives.

6.2 Epidemiology

For patients with nail psoriasis, certain clinical features are more prevalent than others and the majority of these features are found mainly in the fingernails [6]. In a 2012 study, nail pitting was present in the majority of 71 patients who had psoriatic nails; this abnormal variation occurred in the fingernails and/or toenails of 43 (60.6 %) of the patients [7]. Onycholysis was the most common nail bed change which was displayed in the fingernails and/or toenails of 52.1 % of the patients [7]. According to a study by Brazzelli et al., when looking at each individual fingernail, pitting was most commonly seen in the fourth nail of the right hand and the third nail of the left hand [8]. Onycholysis was seen more frequently in the first fingernail (thumb) of the right hand and the fourth on the left hand [8]. Overall, the fourth fingernail and the first toenail were the most affected by psoriatic changes [8]. Pitting in the toenails is relatively rare [8]. Only 2.9 % of patients had pitting in the toenails while 46.0 % had fingernail pitting [8]. On the contrary, in this study, onycholysis was more prevalent in the toenails (68.6 %) than the fingernails (46.0 %) [8].

Additionally, according to a 2011 study conducted in Greece, out of the 225 psoriatic patients, 152 (66.7 %) had psoriasis of the nails [9]. The most prevalent features out of this population were an oil-drop salmon patch discoloration and onycholysis with 79.6 and 76.3 % of the patients displaying these features, respectively [9]. Pitting was found in 57.9 % of the patients, while subungual hyperkeratosis was found in 50.7 % [9]. Crumbling of the nail was found in 41.4 % of the patients [9]. Leukonychia and hemorrhages were apparent in 28.9 % of the patients, and red spots were the least common and only found in two of the patients [9].

Furthermore, a 2007 study from Kuwait demonstrated that the prevalence of nail changes was 37.81 % in children with psoriasis [10]. For these patients with nail implications, nail pitting, the most common feature, was found in 61.84 % of the children, followed by onycholysis in 30.26 % of patients, subungual hyperkeratosis in 13.16 % of patients, and finally discoloration of the nail plate in 7.90 % of the children [10]. When compared to adults, this study shows that a smaller percentage of children with psoriasis have nail changes [10]. However, the order of the frequency of the nail changes including nail pitting, onycholysis, subungual hyperkeratosis, and discoloration of the nail is similar [10].

The distribution of the psoriatic characteristics differs between fingernails and toenails. Toenails typically display discoloration, subungual hyperkeratosis, onycholysis, and crumbling while the fingernails more commonly display pitting, subungual hyperkeratosis, splinter hemorrhages, and oil spots [8, 11]. As can be seen in Table 6.1, there are great variations between different studies in the prevalence of the specific nail features, demonstrating the need for studies that use a greater population of patients with psoriatic nail changes. The table compares fingernail versus toenail involvement of the clinical features. The statistically significant results in Table 6.1 demonstrate that pitting and onycholysis are very common in psoriatic fingernails; studies by Palmou et al., Puri et al., and van der Velden et al. further support this notion (Table 6.2) [3, 12, 13]. In addition, subungual hyperkeratosis and onycholysis are common in the toenails, while pitting and leukonychia are relatively rare in the toenails.

6.3 History

Nail manifestations of psoriasis were first described by Robert Willan in his textbook *On Cutaneous Diseases* published in London in 1808 [14]. Psoriasis was designated as lepra vulgaris. In 1872, Hebra first described nail pitting, and in 1948, John Alkiewicz first identified parakeratosis as the cause of nail pitting [15]. Then, in 2003, the ability to evaluate the clinical features of nail psoriasis improved immensely with the establishment of the Nail Psoriasis Severity Index (NAPSI). NAPSI is a significant tool that enables physicians to determine the severity of nail psoriasis and its response to treatment [16].

6.4 Clinical Features

6.4.1 Overview

The clinical features of nail psoriasis, as well as skin psoriasis, are due to inflammatory hyperkeratotic papules. These papules present differently based on where in the nail they occur (Table 6.3) [5]. The clinical features originate in either the nail matrix or nail bed. The nail matrix is the portion of the nail unit that produces the nail plate. The lunula is the most distal portion of the matrix, which can be seen through the nail plate and appears as a white arch. Conversely, the nail bed is a portion of the nail unit that is situated between the lunula and the hyponychium – the skin underneath the nail plate edge [5, 17].

Nail pitting, leukonychia (white spots), red spots in the lunula, and at times crumbling originate in the nail matrix and become incorporated into the developing nail plate. All of these characteristics are seen in the nail plate. In contrast, onycholysis, splinter hemorrhages, hyperkeratosis, and an "oil-drop" salmon patch

Table 6.1 The prevalence of particular nail changes in fingernails and toenails in patients with psoriatic nails

Nail clinical feature	Percentage of patients with *fingernail* involvement in study by Brazzelli et al. [8]	Percentage of patients with *fingernail* involvement in study by Salomon et al. [11]	Percentage of patients with *fingernail* involvement in study by Idrees et al. [7]	Percentage of patients with *toenail* involvement in study by Brazzelli et al. [8]	Percentage of patients with *toenail* involvement in study by Salomon et al. [11]	Percentage of patients with *toenail* involvement in study by Idrees et al. [7]
Pitting	46.0 %	56.6 %	57.7 %	2.9 %	1.2 %	59.2 %
Leukonychia	5.1 %	N/A	1.4 %	8.0 %	N/A	0.0 %
Crumbling	14.6 %	N/A	N/A	53.3 %	N/A	N/A
Onycholysis	46.0 %	2.4 %[a]	49.3 %	68.6 %	2.4 %[a]	46.5 %
Splinter hemorrhages	24.1 %	N/A	N/A	10.2 %	N/A	N/A
Subungual hyperkeratosis	5.1 %	79.5 %	28.2 %	51.8 %	74.7 %	29.6 %
Discoloration including oil drop	13.9 %	12.0 %	7.0 %	29.2 %	7.2 %	5.6 %

[a]Not statistically significant

Table 6.2 Frequency of specific nail abnormalities in patients with psoriasis

Nail clinical feature	Percentage of patients with nail involvement in study by Palmou et al. [12]	Percentage of patients with nail involvement in study by Puri et al. [13]	Percentage of patients with nail involvement in study by van der Velden et al. [3]
Pitting	65.4 %	70 %	73.5 %
Leukonychia	7.7 %	N/A	40.8 %
Crumbling	9.6 %	N/A	42.9 %
Onycholysis	27.1 %	52 %	93.9 %
Splinter hemorrhages	21.2 %	12 %	93.9 %
Subungual hyperkeratosis	7.7 %	40 %	46.9 %
Discoloration including oil drop	N/A	10 %	67.3 %

Table 6.3 Function of different constituents of the nail apparatus

Constituent	Function
Proximal nail fold (PNF)	Protects the nail matrix from environmental agents. The cuticle, the cornified cell layer of the PNF, helps seal the nail plate and prevents nail matrix damage
Nail matrix	Produces the nail plate. The proximal matrix produces the dorsal nail plate; the distal matrix produces the ventral nail plate
Nail bed	Provides adhesion to the nail plate as its horny layer is part of the ventral nail plate
Hyponychium	Transition zone between the nail bed and the epidermis

Table 6.4 Main clinical features of nail psoriasis in nail matrix and nail bed

Clinical features originating in the nail matrix	Clinical features originating in the nail bed
Nail pitting	Onycholysis
Leukonychia (white spots)	Splinter hemorrhages
Red spots in the lunula	Subungual hyperkeratosis
Crumbling	Oil-drop salmon patch discoloration

discoloration occur in the nail bed (Table 6.4) [16]. Other nail changes in patients with psoriasis include longitudinal ridges, extending from the cuticle to the distal part of the nail, and transverse ridges (Beau lines) [11]. Beau lines are a consequence of sporadic irritation of the nail matrix and may spread to the nail plate, resulting in an impermanent loss of the nail [6].

Aside from the primary clinical features of nail psoriasis, there are often secondary features present as well. For instance, fungal infections (onychomycosis), which can mimic the clinical features of nail psoriasis, were present in 18 % of the patients with psoriatic nails. Unfortunately, the presence of both conditions increases the severity of nail psoriasis [11, 18]. Moreover, there is a significant correlation between psoriatic nails, joint pain, and joint deformities [19]. All of these clinical features are clues to the physician that the patient has nail psoriasis (Fig. 6.1).

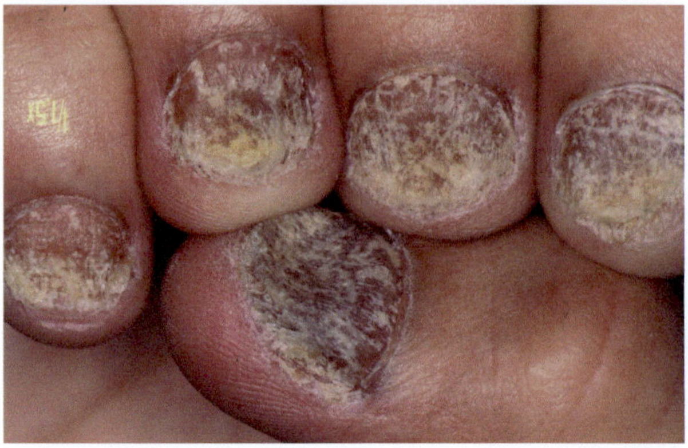

Fig. 6.1 These nails show signs of both nail bed and nail matrix psoriasis: note thickening due to subungual hyperkeratosis, abnormalities of the nail plate surface, leukonychia, and erythema of the lunula

Table 6.5 Descriptions of nail matrix features

Clinical features	Main characteristics
Pitting	Irregular, superficial depressions in the nail plate
Leukonychia	White spots in the nail plate
Red spots in the lunula	The white arch of the nail contains erythematous spots
Crumbling	Destruction of the nail plate

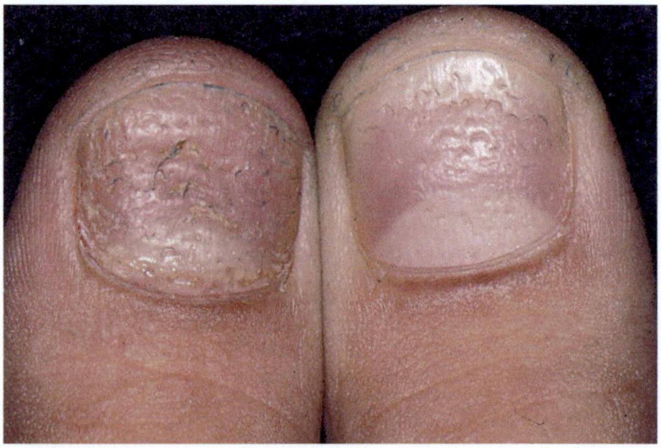

Fig. 6.2 Psoriatic pitting. Pits are large, deep, and irregularly distributed. Onycholysis is also present

6.4.2 Nail Matrix Features

Nail matrix features include pitting, leukonychia, red spots in the lunula, and crumbling (Table 6.5). Nail pits can be recognized as superficial depressions in the nail plate that move distally with nail growth [20, 21]. Pits are typically irregularly spaced and almost exclusively seen in the fingernails with rare occurrence in the toenails [8, 22]. Psoriatic pits are typically deep, large, and irregularly distributed (Fig. 6.2). Nail pits are due to psoriasis of the proximal nail matrix that causes abnormal keratinization with the presence of parakeratotic cells in the uppermost surface of the nail plate [23, 24]. The proximal nail fold can also contribute to the formation of nail pitting [21]. When these loosely packed cells slough off from the nail plate, a pit or depression forms [24]. The remaining parakeratotic cells are visible as scales within the pit [25]. The number of pits is important: less than 20 pits are nonspecific for diagnosis, but the presence of more than 20 pits is suggestive of psoriasis and more than 60 pits is diagnostic [26]. In a 2013 study, none of the patients in the control group (without psoriasis) had more than 20 pits while 8 % of the psoriasis patients had between 20 and 60 pits and 12 % had more than 60 pits. Moreover, the incidence of nail pitting rises with increases in the severity of psoriasis [22]. Nail pitting is characteristic of psoriasis; however, it may also be seen in alopecia areata and eczema [6, 20, 26]. Evaluating the nails for pitting is essential as it can provide support for diagnosing psoriasis [22, 27].

Unlike nail pitting, leukonychia occurs when psoriasis affects the middle and/or distal part of the nail matrix, and the parakeratotic cells are within the ventral nail plate [24]. In leukonychia the nail surface is smooth; persistence of the parakeratotic cells as white scales within the pits may resemble leukonychia, but in this case the nail has a rough surface [5]. The perception of white spots is due to the desquamation of parakeratotic cells and the light reflected on the nail plate [24, 28].

Red spots in the lunula are a result of a modification of the amount of blood beneath the nail due to a variation in the pattern of the vessels, vessel dilatation, or a change in the composition of the blood. There are no signs of an increase in the amount of capillaries or dilation; thus, it is proposed that the erythematous lunulae are due to either augmented arteriolar blood flow or venous vasodilation of unclear origin [29]. Furthermore, alterations in the nail plate may result in a greater appearance of the underlying nail bed or a lack of compression of the blood vessels in the nail bed [29, 30]. In particular, a decrease in the thickness of the nail plate may present with nail bed erythema [31]. Moreover, the lunula may look spotted or red with intermediate and ventral matrix involvement [32].

Nail crumbling, another nail matrix feature, is related to a thick and dystrophic nail plate as well as a hyperkeratotic nail bed [33]. The consequences of crumbling sometimes include a visible comprehensive devastation of the nail plate [33]. Crumbling may be present when extensive psoriatic changes affect the entire nail matrix [28]. Additionally, crumbling is suggestive of a long duration of disease [5].

6.4.3 Nail Bed Features

Nail bed features include onycholysis, splinter hemorrhages, subungual hyperkeratosis, and oil-drop salmon patch discoloration (Table 6.6). Onycholysis appears white due to the loss of attachment of the nail plate to the nail bed [20]. The detachment is due to a significant lesion at the hyponychium where parakeratosis interferes with the adhesion of the nail plate to the nail bed [20, 24]. As a result, onycholysis is frequently associated with keratin fragments that accumulate below the nail plate [24]. Onycholysis usually originates distally and/or laterally and

Table 6.6 Descriptions of nail bed features

Clinical features	Main characteristics
Onycholysis	Detachment of the nail plate from the nail bed
Splinter hemorrhages	Ruptured nail capillary producing a dark red longitudinal line
Subungual hyperkeratosis	An accumulation of keratinocytes below the nail plate
Oil-drop salmon patch discoloration	A yellow/reddish-brown plaque with excessive glycoproteins

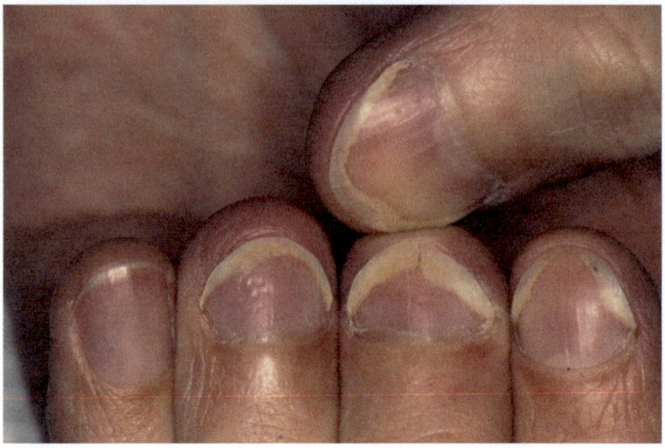

Fig. 6.3 Onycholysis without erythematous border. Diagnosis is suggested by presence of irregular pits in some nails

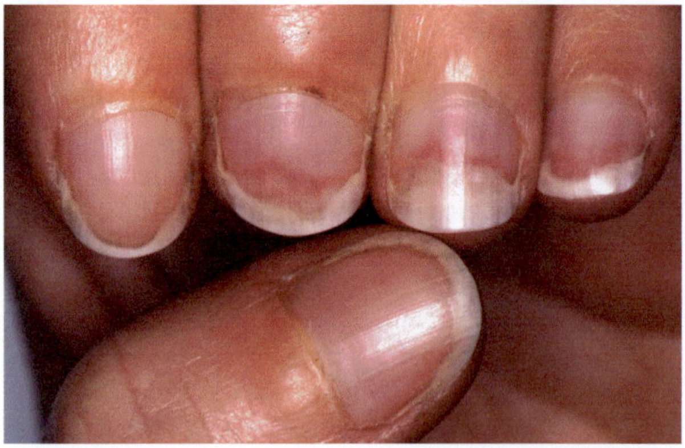

Fig. 6.4 Onycholysis with erythematous border

advances proximally toward the nail matrix [5, 34]. This separation occurs along a convex line [6]. Air accumulates underneath the nail plate and is responsible for the whitish appearance (Fig. 6.3) [35]. An erythematous border around the onycholytic area is diagnostic for psoriasis and most frequently seen in fingernails (Fig. 6.4) [36]. Onycholysis in combination with subungual hyperkeratosis is typical for psoriatic toenails [36]. Trauma and irritation also have the potential to cause

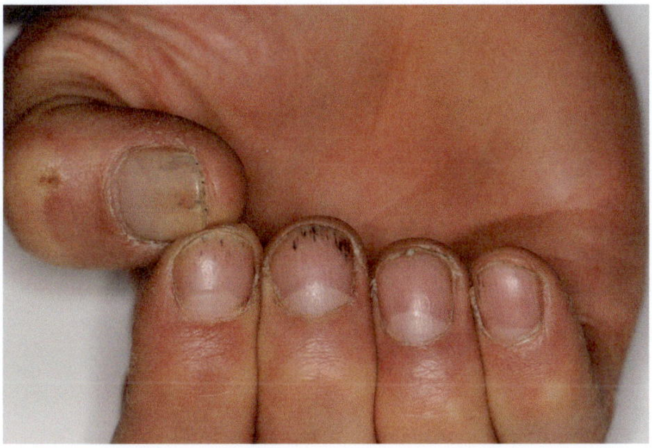

Fig. 6.5 Distal splinter hemorrhages. The clinical features are suggestive but not diagnostic. In this patient diagnosis was confirmed by presence of typical scalp psoriasis

onycholysis. Bacteria and yeast may invade more easily in the presence of onycholysis, and discoloration may ensue [21]. For instance, a greenish or brown color may occur due to the infiltration of *Pseudomonas aeruginosa*, mold, or yeast [34]. Interestingly, nails affected by onycholysis have a faster growth rate than unaffected nails; however, the etiology of this phenomenon remains unclear [37]. Unfortunately during prolonged onycholysis, abnormal keratinization of the nail bed as a result of environmental exposure reduces the likelihood that the nail plate will be able to reattach to the nail bed [21].

Splinter hemorrhages also involve the nail bed and are longitudinal dark red lines (1–3 mm in length) that occur when the capillaries in the dermal papillae rupture (Fig. 6.5) [20, 38]. Capillary rupture is due to excessive inflammation and swelling or clots [39]. The anatomy of the nail bed capillaries is the foundation for the characteristic appearance of splinter hemorrhages, and the hemorrhages' longitudinal path also follows the direction of nail growth. The papillary network contains arterioles, which originate from deeper vessels that anastomose and form an arcade. Arterioles extend from the arcade into the dermis's papillae to form capillary loops which drain into the venules parallel to the arterioles [40]. Most of the capillary loops occur in the distal third of the nail [39]. According to an Austrian study with 120 participants, there is an average of 8.71 capillaries/mm in the nail bed. A hairpin structure with a linear afferent and efferent portion connected by a rounded end point is the normal morphology of these capillaries, residing in the dermal ridges of the nail bed [41, 42].

Another nail bed feature is subungual hyperkeratosis, which is an accumulation of scales beneath the nail plate [20]. Subungual hyperkeratosis involves the distal nail bed and hyponychium [24]. In the fingernails, scaly debris gather under the nail plate [24]. In the toenails, however, subungual hyperkeratosis is normally securely attached to the thickened nail plate [43]. Subungual hyperkeratosis can differ in its clinical appearance due to differences in color and the amount of keratosis [5]. In psoriasis, subungual hyperkeratosis is usually silvery white (Fig. 6.6), but may be

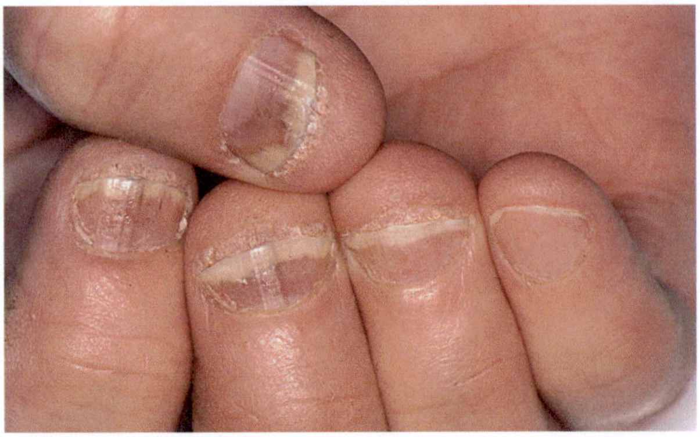

Fig. 6.6 Severe subungual hyperkeratosis. The silvery white color is typical for nail psoriasis

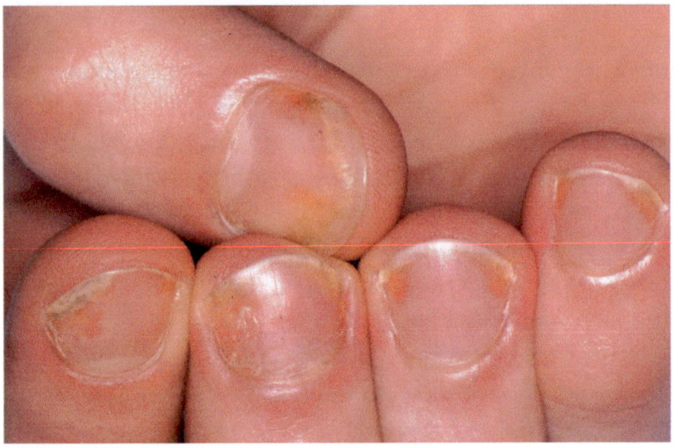

Fig. 6.7 Salmon patches and onycholysis with erythematous border. Note pits with scaly surface on the third fingernail

yellow and greasy, or green or brown if there is secondary colonization [5]. Pathology shows thickening of the stratum corneum, parakeratosis, and loss of the granular layer in the hyponychium [5]. The yellow-greasy appearance is due to the accumulation of serum glycoprotein, and the green or brown color is due to the colonization of various microorganisms [5]. Clinicians can identify the severity of psoriatic activity in the hyponychium based on the degree of elevation of the nail plate above the nail bed [5].

The oil-drop salmon patch discoloration is a yellow/reddish-brown drop that occurs in the nail bed and/or the hyponychium and is seen by observation through the translucent nail plate [35]. These salmon patches are irregular in size and shape [6]. The oil drop may be seen in the central part of the nail, or it may surround an onycholytic area in the distal nail bed (Fig. 6.7) [43]. Psoriatic inflammation involving dilated capillaries, the infiltration of lymphocytes, parakeratotic cells, and neutrophils contribute to the salmon spots [24, 35]. The characteristic salmon color can be further explained by the overlying nail plate, which obstructs air from going in between the keratin layers and results in a coherent appearance [44]. Moreover, the oil-drop sign is due to a subungual accrual of glycoprotein [24].

6.5 Diagnostic Clues

Clinical diagnosis of nail psoriasis can be difficult as the symptoms are common features of many nail disorders. The presence of multiple signs in different nails is highly suggestive. Diagnosis is particularly difficult in the case of simple onycholysis (onycholysis without peripheral oil-drop discoloration) in the fingernails and in the case of subungual hyperkeratosis occurring in fingernails and/or toenails. For simple onycholysis, not associated with other nail signs of psoriasis, dermoscopy of the hyponychium is probably the only way to make the correct diagnosis. In the instance of subungual hyperkeratosis, the presence of white silvery scales is highly suggestive of psoriasis. Furthermore, acquired subungual hyperkeratosis involving all nails, all fingernails, or all toenails is very suggestive. Other suggestive features of nail psoriasis include more than 20 irregular pits in the fingernails, onycholysis with an erythematous border, and salmon patches in the nail bed.

Summary for the Clinician

In summary, it is essential for clinicians to be able to recognize the wide array of nail matrix and nail bed features in order to diagnose nail psoriasis and to be aware of other potential complications that may arise [3]. For example, the clinical changes in psoriatic nails can increase the risk of infection. A fungal infection with nail psoriasis will worsen the disorder; therefore, it is vital for the clinician to exclude their coexistence [18]. Additionally, many patients with nail psoriasis also present with psoriatic arthritis. By recognizing this significant correlation, physicians have the ability to reduce the severity of any current or future joint involvement related to psoriasis [19]. Moreover, the overall quality of life is significantly diminished in patients with nail involvement compared to those without. Patients with psoriatic nails tend to have a larger area of their skin affected by psoriasis and take more days off of work, and their overall health is worse than patients without nail features [45]. Therefore, identifying the clinical features of nail psoriasis and treating the symptoms is essential for the well-being of the patient.

References

1. Calvert HT, Smith MA, Wells RS. Psoriasis and the nails. Br J Dermatol. 1963;75:415–8.
2. De Jong EMGJ, Seegers BAMPA, Gulinck MK, Boezeman JBM, van de Kerkhof PCM. Psoriasis of the nails associated with disability in a large number of patients: results of a recent interview with 1,728 patients. Dermatology. 1996;193(4):300–3. doi:10.1159/000246274.
3. van der Velden HM, Klaassen KM, van de Kerkhof PC, Pasch MC. Fingernail psoriasis reconsidered: a case-control study. J Am Acad Dermatol. 2013;69(2):245–52. doi:10.1016/j.jaad.2013.02.009.
4. Cannavo SP, Guarneri F, Vaccaro M, Borgia F, Guarneri B. Treatment of psoriatic nails with topical cyclosporin: a prospective, randomized placebo-controlled study. Dermatology. 2003;206(2):153–6, 68469.
5. Zaias N. Psoriasis of the nail: a clinical-pathologic study. Arch Dermatol. 1969;99(5):567–79. doi:10.1001/archderm.1969.01610230059011.

6. Baran R, Tosti A. Nails. In: Fitzpatrick TB, Freedberg IM, editors. Fitzpatrick's dermatology in general medicine, vol. I. 6th ed. New York: McGraw-Hill, Medical Pub. Division; 2003.
7. Idrees S, Uddin R, Rizvi SDA, Tahir M. Frequency of nail changes in psoriasis. J Pak Assoc Dermatol. 2012;22(4):315–9.
8. Brazzelli V, Carugno A, Alborghetti A, Grasso V, Cananzi R, Fornara L, De Silvestri A, Borroni G. Prevalence, severity and clinical features of psoriasis in fingernails and toenails in adult patients: Italian experience. J Eur Acad Dermatol Venereol. 2012;26(11):1354–9. doi:10.1111/j.1468-3083.2011.04289.x.
9. Kyriakou A, Patsatsi A, Sotiriadis D. Detailed analysis of specific nail psoriasis features and their correlations with clinical parameters: a cross-sectional study. Dermatology. 2011;223(3): 222–9. doi:10.1159/000332974.
10. Al-Mutairi N, Manchanda Y, Nour-Eldin O. Nail changes in childhood psoriasis: a study from Kuwait. Pediatr Dermatol. 2007;24(1):7–10. doi:10.1111/j.1525-1470.2007.00324.x.
11. Salomon J, Szepietowski JC, Proniewicz A. Psoriatic nails: a prospective clinical study. J Cutan Med Surg. 2003;7(4):317–21. doi:10.1007/s10227-002-0143-0.
12. Palmou N, Marzo-Ortega H, Ash Z, Goodfield M, Coates LC, Helliwell PS, McGonagle D. Linear pitting and splinter haemorrhages are more commonly seen in the nails of patients with established psoriasis in comparison to psoriatic arthritis. Dermatology. 2011;223(4):370–3. doi:10.1159/000335571.
13. Puri N, Mahajan BB. Nail changes in psoriasis – a profile. J Pak Assoc Dermatol. 2011; 21(3):165–9.
14. Levell N. Robert Willan. In: Löser C, Plewig G, Burgdorf W, editors. Pantheon of dermatology: outstanding historical figures. 1st ed. Berlin: Springer; 2013. p. 1188–93.
15. Alkiewicz J. Psoriasis of the nails. Br J Dermatol Syph. 1948;60(6):195–200.
16. Rich P, Scher RK. Nail Psoriasis Severity Index: a useful tool for evaluation of nail psoriasis. J Am Acad Dermatol. 2003;49(2):206–12.
17. Zaias N. Embryology of the human nail. Arch Dermatol. 1963;87(1):37–53. doi:10.1001/archderm.1963.01590130043010.
18. Kacar N. The prevalence, aetiological agents and therapy of onychomycosis in patients with psoriasis: a prospective controlled trial. Clin Exp Dermatol. 2007;32(1):1–5.
19. Elkayam O, Ophir J, Yaron M, Caspi D. Psoriatic arthritis: interrelationships between skin and joint manifestations related to onset, course and distribution. Clin Rheumatol. 2000;19(4): 301–5.
20. Edwards F, de Berker D. Nail psoriasis: clinical presentation and best practice recommendations. Drugs. 2009;69(17):2351–61.
21. Jadhav VM, Mahajan PM, Mhaske CB. Nail pitting and onycholysis. Indian J Dermatol Venereol Leprol. 2009;75(6):631–3. doi:10.4103/0378-6323.57740.
22. Singh SK. Finger nail pitting in psoriasis and its relation with different variables. Indian J Dermatol. 2013;58(4):310–2. doi:10.4103/0019-5154.113955.
23. Zaias N. The nail in health and disease. 2nd ed. Norwalk: Appleton & Lange; 1990.
24. Holzberg M. Common nail disorders. Dermatol Clin. 2006;24(3):349–54. doi:10.1016/j.det.2006.03.001.
25. Pinkus H, Mehregan AH. The primary histologic lesion of seborrheic dermatitis and psoriasis. J Invest Dermatol. 1966;46(1):109–16.
26. Baran R, Dawber RPR. Baran and Dawber's diseases of the nails and their management. 3rd ed. Malden: Blackwell Science; 2001.
27. Freedberg IM, Fitzpatrick TB. Fitzpatrick's dermatology in general medicine. 5th ed. New York: McGraw-Hill, Health Professions Division; 1999.
28. Baran R, Dawber RPR. Diseases of the nails and their management. Cambridge, MA: Blackwell Scientific Publications; 1984.
29. Wilkerson MG, Wilkin JK. Red lunulae revisited: a clinical and histopathologic examination. J Am Acad Dermatol. 1989;20(3):453–7.
30. de Berker D. Erythronychia. Dermatol Ther. 2012;25(6):603–11. doi:10.1111/j.1529-8019.2012.01525.x.

31. Lesher Jr JL, Peterson CM, Lane JE. An unusual case of factitious onychodystrophy. Pediatr Dermatol. 2004;21(3):239–41. doi:10.1111/j.0736-8046.2004.21310.x.
32. Jiaravuthisan MM, Sasseville D, Vender RB, Murphy F, Muhn CY. Psoriasis of the nail: anatomy, pathology, clinical presentation, and a review of the literature on therapy. J Am Acad Dermatol. 2007;57(1):1–27. doi:10.1016/j.jaad.2005.07.073.
33. Baran R, Dawber RPR, Haneke E, Tosti A, Bristow I. A text atlas of nail disorders: techniques in investigation and diagnosis. 3rd ed. London: Martin Dunitz; 2003.
34. Daniel 3rd CR, Iorizzo M, Piraccini BM, Tosti A. Grading simple chronic paronychia and onycholysis. Int J Dermatol. 2006;45(12):1447–8. doi:10.1111/j.1365-4632.2006.03128.x.
35. Kouskoukis CE, Scher RK, Ackerman AB. The "oil drop" sign of psoriatic nails. Am J Dermatopathol. 1983;5(3):259–62. doi:10.1097/00000372-198306000-00012.
36. Tosti A, Piraccini B. Chapter 89: Biology of nails and nail disorders. In: Wolff K, editor. Fitzpatrick's dermatology in general medicine. New York: McGraw-Hill; 2012.
37. Dawber RP, Samman PD, Bottoms E. Fingernail growth in idiopathic and psoriatic onycholysis. Br J Dermatol. 1971;85(6):558–60.
38. Jackson RH. Splinter haemorrhages in the finger nails. Br Med J. 1963;2(5371):1485–6.
39. Kilpatrick ZM, Greenberg PA, Sanford JP. Splinter hemorrhages – their clinical significance. Arch Intern Med. 1965;115:730–5.
40. Wolfram-Gabel R, Sick H. Vascular networks of the periphery of the fingernail. J Hand Surg Br. 1995;20(4):488–92.
41. Hoerth C, Kundi M, Katzenschlager R, Hirschl M. Qualitative and quantitative assessment of nailfold capillaries by capillaroscopy in healthy volunteers. Vasa. 2012;41(1):19–26. doi:10.1024/0301-1526/a000159.
42. Zaiac MN, Weiss E. Mohs micrographic surgery of the nail unit and squamous cell carcinoma. Dermatol Surg. 2001;27(3):246–51.
43. Tosti A, Piraccini B. Dermatological diseases that affect the nail. In: Hordinsky MK, Sawaya M, Scher RK, editors. Atlas of hair and nails. Philadelphia: Saunders; 2000. p. xii, 252 p.
44. Haneke E. Non-infectious inflammatory disorders of the nail apparatus. J Dtsch Dermatol Ges. 2009;7(9):787–97. doi:10.1111/j.1610-0387.2009.07037.x.
45. Radtke MA, Langenbruch AK, Schafer I, Herberger K, Reich K, Augustin M. Nail psoriasis as a severity indicator: results from the PsoReal study. Patient Relat Outcome Meas. 2011;2:1–6. doi:10.2147/PROM.S14861.

Ultrasound Imaging of Psoriatic Nails

7

Ximena Wortsman and Rosamary Soto

Contents

Key Features

- Ultrasound can provides exquisite detail of the nail anatomy, covering the ungual and periungual regions.
- This technique recognizes submillimeter lesions and can show the ungual blood flow in real time.
- Ultrasound is capable of detecting subclinical changes in psoriasis.
- Psoriatic onychopathy may show a variable appearance according to the phase of the disease.

X. Wortsman, MD (✉)
Department of Radiology and Department of Dermatology, Institute for Diagnostic Imaging and Research of the Skin and Soft Tissue, Clinica Servet, Faculty of Medicine, University of Chile, Lo Fontecilla 201, of 734, Las Condes, Santiago, RM, Chile
e-mail: xworts@yahoo.com, xwo@tie.cl

R. Soto, MD
Department of Dermatology, Faculty of Medicine, University of Chile, Santos Dumont 999, Independencia, Santiago, RM, Chile
e-mail: rosamary_soto@hotmail.com

D. Rigopoulos, A. Tosti (eds.), *Nail Psoriasis: From A to Z*,
DOI 10.1007/978-3-319-08810-5_7

- Common sonographic signs going from early to late phases are: thickening of the nail bed, loss of definition of the ventral plate, focal hyperechoic deposits in the ventral plate (commonly subclinical), thickening and loss of definition of the dorsal and ventral plates, and thickened, wavy plates sometimes with posterior an acoustic shadowing artifact.
- The assessment of activity may also be performed by tracking the vascularity on color or power Doppler.
- Hypervascularity in the nail bed is frequently found during the active phases of the disease.
- Enthesopathy (i.e. decreased echogenicity) of the distal insertion of the extensor tendon and subclinical anechoic fluid in the joints may also be detected during nail ultrasound examinations.
- Ultrasound can be a potent adjunct tool in the early diagnosis and monitoring of psoriatic onychopathy.

7.1 Introduction

Psoriasis is a common disease in dermatologic practice that affects approximately 2 % of the population, with a rising incidence over the years [1]. Nail involvement has long been recognized as a common manifestation of psoriasis, occurring in up to 50 % of patients [2] with an estimated lifetime incidence of 80–90 %. Nail psoriasis occurs more frequently in patients with severe disease such as those with psoriatic arthritis, with a prevalence of 70–80 % in this latter group [3].

However, nail psoriasis also occurs in 40 % of patients with mild psoriasis (PASI ≤10). In patients with moderate to severe psoriasis, approximately 82 % have nail psoriasis symptoms [4]. Importantly, between 1 and 5 % of patients have affected nails without skin lesions [5]. Biopsies are difficult to perform in nails since they may leave permanent cosmetic sequels; therefore, to have at our disposal a noninvasive window to unveil the anatomic details of the nail unit and their pathologies would be of great benefit.

Ultrasound has been increasingly used for studying skin and nails lesions and has become a daily imaging technique in our practice. Furthermore, the addition of variable frequency ultrasound to the clinical dermatologic practice has been reported to increase the correctness of the diagnosis from 73 to 97 % [6]. This method of imaging provides exquisite detail of the nail anatomy, covering from the surface of the ungual plate to the bony margin of the distal phalanx. It can recognize submillimeter lesions and can show the ungual blood flow in real time [7–9]. To date this anatomical information is not completely provided by other imaging modalities such as confocal microscopy (CFM), optical coherence tomography (OCT), or magnetic resonance imaging (MRI). For example, CFM and OCT present very low penetration and do not give information on vascularity. Currently, the commercially available MRI machines have low resolution and have problems detecting ungual tumors that measure ≤3 mm [7]. The limitations of variable frequency ultrasound are the detection of pigments, lesions that measure ≤0.1 mm, and epidermal-only lesions, but it gives us a wide range of possibilities for studying nail conditions [6].

Thus, the usage of sonography for studying nails has been growing fast, and nowadays reports in the literature include a wide spectrum of common ungual tumors and pseudotumors, congenital conditions, inflammatory diseases, and cosmetic alterations, among other conditions [7–10].

In psoriasis, ultrasound has been used for supporting early diagnosis and monitoring the involvement in the five most common targets that are affected by the disease: joints, tendons, entheses (i.e., insertion of tendons), skin, and nails [11]. Moreover, this imaging technique is capable of detecting subclinical changes in psoriasis [12]. The nail has been also considered as a specialized enthesis, considering the histologic disposition of the distal insertion of the branches of the lateral bands of the extensor tendon that tend to embrace the nail unit [13]. Therefore, the pathologies that affect the distal interphalangeal joint and the enthesis of the extensor tendon may commonly affect the morphology and functioning of the nail.

7.2 Technical Considerations and Normal Sonographic Anatomy of the Nail

This technique requires multichannel ultrasound machines that work with variable frequency probes with an upper frequency that commonly ranges between 15 and 22 MHz. The usage of compact linear probes (hockey stick shaped) is recommended because they present a better adaptation to the surface and size of the nail. A copious amount of gel is applied over the nail and periungual regions with the fingers or toes in the fully extended position. It is also suggested that comparative studies be performed, side by side (e.g., right to left or medial to lateral) to more easily recognize the abnormalities [7–10]. The normal sonographic anatomy of the nail unit includes three parts: the nail bed, the nail plate, and the periungual tissue. The nail bed includes the matrix region in its proximal part. On ultrasound, the ungual plates show as bilaminar and parallel hyperechoic structures (dorsal and ventral plates) with a hypoechoic virtual interplate space in between the plates. This space tends to show as slightly more hyperechoic on higher frequencies (≥20 MHz). The ungual bed appears as a hypoechoic tissue beneath the ungual plates (Fig. 7.1). On color or

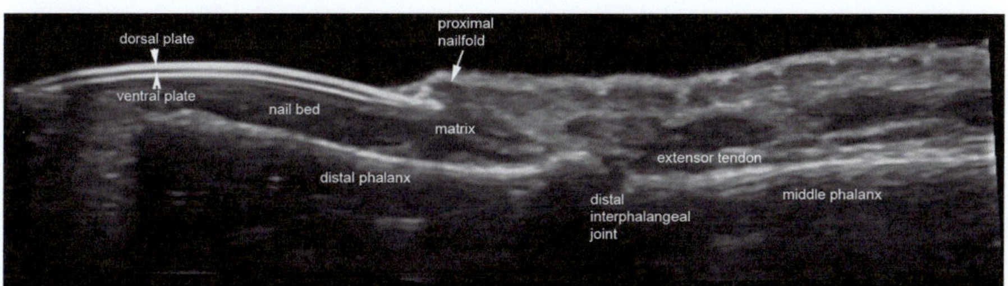

Fig. 7.1 Normal ultrasound anatomy of the nail (gray scale, longitudinal view)

power (i.e., detection of slow flow) Doppler, it is possible to detect the vascularity, define the type of vessel (arterial or venous), and measure the velocity (cm/sec) of the nail blood flow in real time. Underlying the nail bed it is possible to detect the hyperechoic and linear bony margin of the distal phalanx. The periungual region can be separated into the lateral and proximal nail folds, and they show the same echostructure already described for the non-glabrous skin with the exception that they lack hypoechoic fatty tissue. Nevertheless, hypoechoic fatty tissue is prominent in the pulp of the fingers. The distal insertion of the lateral bands of the extensor tendon appears as hyperechoic fibrillar structures that show an anisotropy artifact (i.e., they become dark on the screen when the insertion angle is less than 90°). In some extended views of the nail, the anechoic space of the distal interphalangeal joint can also be observed. Usually, 2D views and 3D reconstructions (5–8 s sweeps) which cover all axes of the nail [14, 15] are performed during nail examinations.

7.3 Ultrasound Characteristics of Psoriatic Nails

Psoriatic onychopathy may show a variable appearance according to the phase of the disease. The common sonographic signs in psoriatic nails going from early to late phases are thickening of the nail bed, loss of definition of the ventral plate, focal hyperechoic deposits in the ventral plate (commonly subclinical), thickening and loss of definition of the dorsal and ventral plates, and thickened, wavy plates sometimes with posterior and acoustic shadowing artifact [7–12] (Figs. 7.2 and 7.3). The assessment of activity may also be performed by tracking the vascularity on color or power Doppler. Hypervascularity in the nail bed is frequently found during the active phases of the disease [10, 11, 15] (Fig. 7.4). According to the literature the distance from the ventral plate to the bony margin of the distal phalanx (nail bed thickness) is significantly increased in psoriatic patients when compared with healthy controls. This has been studied in the right index finger – mean 3.0 mm in psoriatic patients (range 2.04–4.01 mm) and mean 1.5 mm in healthy controls (range 1.33–1.79 mm) [12]. Other researchers have reported that the nail bed is 0.5 mm (range 0.3–1.9 mm) significantly thicker in psoriatic patients in comparison with healthy subjects [16]. The increased nail plate and bed thickness have been also described as subclinical [17]. Another interesting feature is the common presence of enthesopathy (i.e., decreased echogenicity) of the distal insertion of the extensor tendon in psoriatic patients [18]. Significant subclinical anechoic fluid in the joints has been reported in psoriatic patients in comparison with healthy controls; this may also be detected during nail ultrasound examinations [17]. These key ultrasound characteristics of psoriatic onychopathy can support both the diagnosis and follow-up phases and demonstrate objective anatomical changes that can also be used in clinical trials. Importantly, this information is obtained noninvasively [19].

Fig. 7.2 Psoriatic onychopathy ultrasound patterns (gray scale, longitudinal views). Thickening of the nail bed (*white vertical line* and *markers*), focal hyperechoic deposit in the ventral plate (*arrow pointing up*), loss of definition of the ventral plate (*arrowhead*), wavy nail plates with posterior acoustic shadowing artifact (*arrows pointing down*)

Psoriatic onychopathy ultrasound patterns

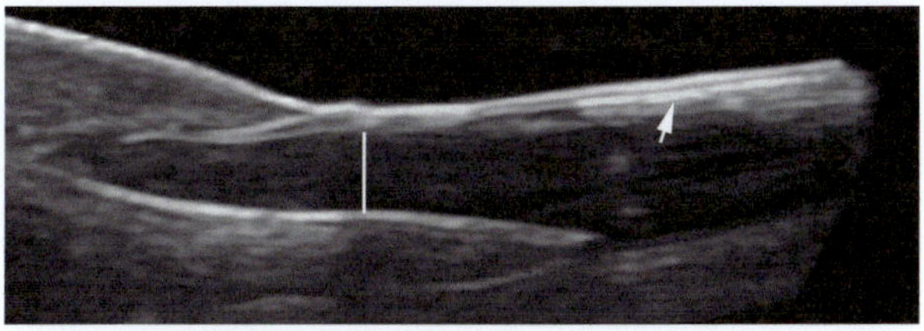

Slight thickening of the nail bed and focal hyperechoic deposit in the ventral plate

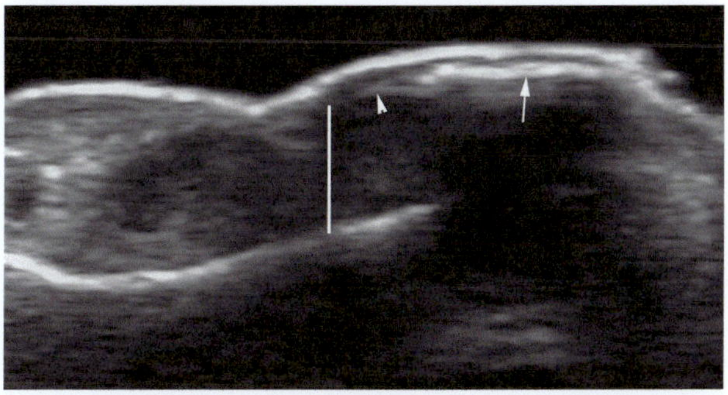

Thickening of the nail bed, loss of definition of the ventral plate and hyperechoic deposit in the ventral plate

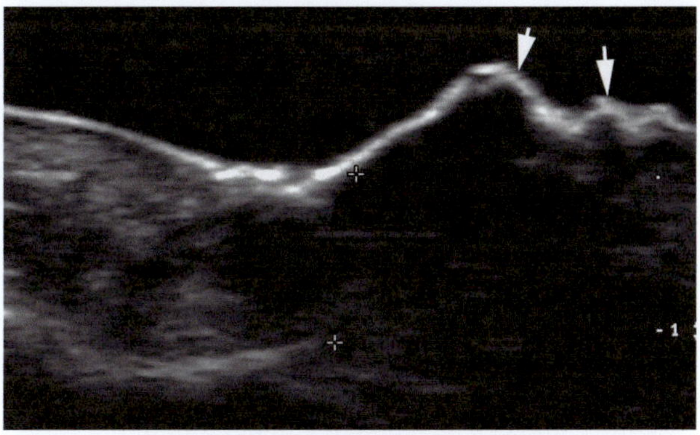

Pronounced thickening of the nail bed, loss of definition of dorsal and ventral plates, wavy nail plates with posterior acoustic shadowing

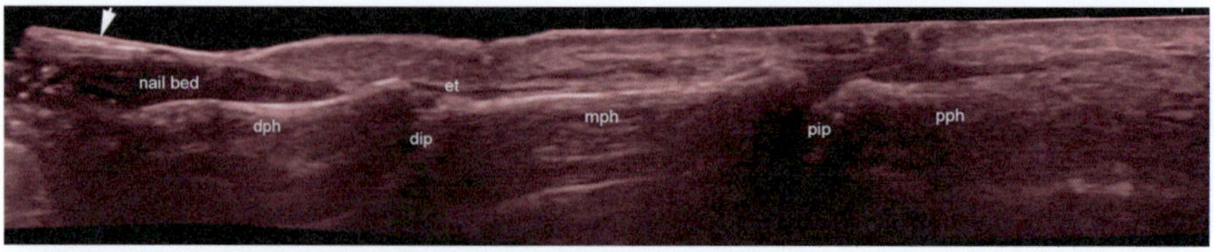

Fig. 7.3 Psoriatic onychopathy extended ultrasound image (gray scale, longitudinal panoramic view, color filter) demonstrates hyperechoic deposit (*arrow*) in the ventral plate. The extended field of view shows the whole finger including the insertion of the extensor tendon (*et*), the distal (*dip*) and proximal (*pip*) interphalangeal joints, as well as the distal (*dph*), middle (*mph*), and proximal (*pph*) phalanges

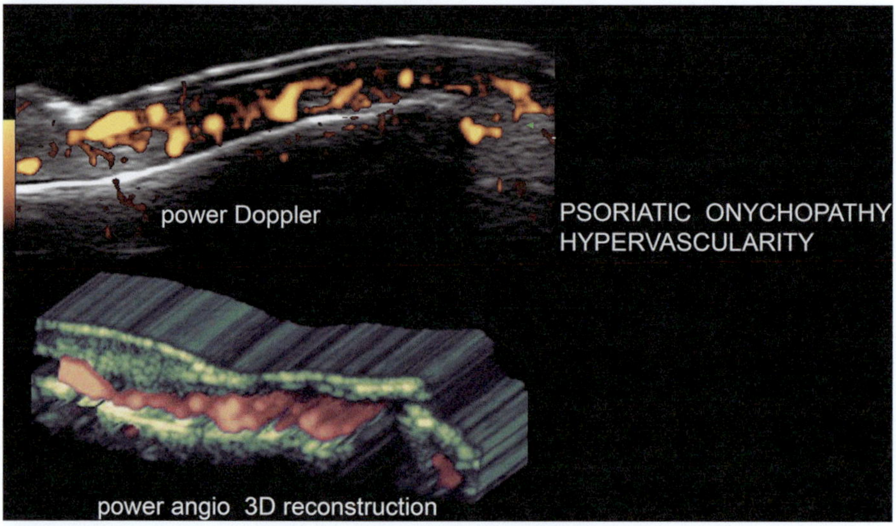

Fig. 7.4 Psoriatic onychopathy hypervascularity during the active phase of the disease

Conclusion

Ultrasound can be a potent adjunct tool in the early diagnosis and monitoring of psoriatic onychopathy.

References

1. Icen M, Crowson CS, McEvoy MT, et al. Trends in incidence of adult-onset psoriasis over three decades; a population-based study. J Am Acad Dermatol. 2009;60:394–401.
2. Jiaravuthisan MM, Sasseville D, Vender RB, et al. Psoriasis of the nail: anatomy, pathology, clinical presentation, and a review of the literature on therapy. J Am Acad Dermatol. 2007;57:1–27.
3. Williamson L, Dalbeth N, Dockerty JL, et al. Extended report: nail disease in psoriatic arthritis – clinically important, potentially treatable and often overlooked. Rheumatology. 2004;43:790–4.

4. Rich P, Griffiths CEM, Reich K, et al. Baseline nail disease in patients with moderate to severe psoriasis and response to treatment with infliximab during 1 year. J Am Acad Dermatol. 2008;58:224–31.
5. Van Laborde S, Scher RK. Developments in the treatment of nail psoriasis, melanonychia striata, and onychomycosis. A review of the literature. Dermatol Clin. 2000;18:37–46.
6. Wortsman X, Wortsman J. Clinical usefulness of variable frequency ultrasound in localized lesions of the skin. J Am Acad Dermatol. 2010;62:247–56.
7. Wortsman X, Wortsman J, Soto R, Saavedra T, Honeyman J, Sazunic I, Corredoira Y. Benign tumors and pseudotumors of the nail: a novel application of sonography. J Ultrasound Med. 2010;29:803–16.
8. Wortsman X, Jemec GBE. Ultrasound imaging of nails. Dermatol Clin. 2006;24:323–8.
9. Thomas L, Vaudaine M, Wortsman X, Jemec GBE, Drapé JL. Imaging the nail unit. In: Baran R, de Berker D, Holzberg M, Thomas L, editors. Baran & Dawber's diseases of the nails and their management. 4th ed. Chichester/West Sussex: Wiley; 2012. p. 132–53.
10. Wortsman X. Sonography of the nail. In: Wortsman X, Jemec GBE, editors. Dermatologic ultrasound with clinical and histologic correlations. New York: Springer; 2013. p. 419–76.
11. Gutierrez M, Filippucci E, De Angelis R, Filosa G, Kane D, Grassi W. A sonographic spectrum of psoriatic arthritis: "the five targets". Clin Rheumatol. 2010;29:133–42.
12. Wortsman X, Holm EA, Jemec GBE, et al. 15 MHz high resolution ultrasound examination of psoriatic nails, (Ultrasonido de alta resolucion de 15 MHz en el estudio de la uña psoriatica). Revista Chilena de Radiología. 2004;10:6–9.
13. McGonagle D, Tan AL, Benjamin M. The biomechanical link between skin and joint disease in psoriasis and psoriatic arthritis: what every dermatologist needs to know. Ann Rheum Dis. 2008;67:1–4.
14. Wortsman X. Common applications of dermatologic sonography. J Ultrasound Med. 2012; 31:97–111.
15. Wortsman X. Ultrasound in dermatology: why, how and when? Semin Ultrasound CT MR. 2013;34:177–95.
16. Aydin SZ, Castillo-Gallego C, Ash ZR, et al. Ultrasonographic assessment of nail in psoriatic disease shows a link between onychopathy and distal interphalangeal joint extensor tendon enthesopathy. Dermatology. 2012;225:231–5.
17. Gisondi P, Idolazzi L, Girolomoni G. Ultrasonography reveals nail thickening in patients with chronic plaque psoriasis. Arch Dermatol Res. 2012;304:727–32.
18. Naredo E, Möller I, de Miguel E, et al., Ultrasound School of the Spanish Society of Rheumatology and Spanish ECO-APs Group. High prevalence of ultrasonographic synovitis and enthesopathy in patients with psoriasis without psoriatic arthritis: a prospective case-control study. Rheumatology (Oxford). 2011;50:1838–48.
19. Gutierrez M, Di Geso L, Salaffi F, Bertolazzi C, Tardella M, Filosa G, Filippucci E, Grassi W. Development of a preliminary US power Doppler composite score for monitoring treatment in PsA. Rheumatology (Oxford). 2012;51:1261–8.

Dermoscopy of Nail Psoriasis

8

Shailee Patel and Antonella Tosti

Contents

Key Features

- Dermoscopy is a noninvasive and quick technique that allows optimal visualization of morphological features of the skin and nails.
- Recently, dermoscopy has been gaining popularity as a regularly utilized tool in managing patients with nail disorders.
- Dermoscopy can help identify diagnostic features such as pitting and salmon patches around onycholysis.
- Dermoscopy can allow diagnosis of nail psoriasis in patients with simple onycholysis or isolated nail bed hyperkeratosis by visualization of twisted capillaries in the hyponychium.
- Dermoscopy can also help monitor response to treatment by changes in capillary density of the hyponychium.

S. Patel, BS • A. Tosti, MD (✉)
Department of Dermatology and Cutaneous Surgery,
University of Miami Miller School of Medicine,
Miami, FL, USA
e-mail: antonella.tosti@unibo.it

D. Rigopoulos, A. Tosti (eds.), *Nail Psoriasis: From A to Z*,
DOI 10.1007/978-3-319-08810-5_8

8.1 Introduction

Dermoscopy is a noninvasive and inexpensive method of magnifying in vivo examination of skin and nails allowing for immediate visualization of specific characteristics that could otherwise be overlooked by the naked eye [1]. Dermoscopy, also known as dermatoscopy, surface microscopy, or epiluminescence microscopy, can evaluate the various structures of nails, such as the nail matrix, nail plate, nail bed, hyponychium, proximal nail fold, and distal edge of the nail plate [2]. Dermoscopy of the nails has been also named onychoscopy [3]. Nail psoriasis has a significant disease burden that is difficult to treat and can cause serious deformities which can lead to chronic dystrophy [4]. Dermoscopy can be valuable in providing better detection of common abnormalities associated with particular diseases, directing management, and assessing response to treatment [1, 5].

8.2 Epidemiology

There is very limited literature on dermoscopy of nail psoriasis. To our knowledge, seven articles or book chapters have been published on the topic [1, 2, 4–8].

8.3 History

In the last 20 years, dermoscopy has enhanced the diagnostic precision of pigmented skin disorders and, more recently, the assessment of nonpigmented skin lesions and diseases of the nail [1, 2]. Dermoscopy is becoming more routinely used to evaluate nail disorders, such as nail psoriasis, as a crucial, inexpensive, and basic tool in clinical practice [1, 7]. Most common dermoscopes have 10× magnification and are made of magnifying optics and a polarized or nonpolarized light source [9]. Normally, most of the light that is exposed to the skin surface reflects back due to the higher refractive index of the stratum corneum (RI 1.55) compared to the refractive index of air (RI 1.0) [10]. Nonpolarized dermoscopes reduce this reflection and increase light penetration by using an interface solution on the surface of the glass plate corresponding the refractive index with the stratum corneum (RI 1.52) and minimizing the air interface [11], whereas polarized dermoscopes exploit two orthogonal filters to cross-polarize light to reduce the reflection. By passing nonpolarized light through a polarizing filter, the emerging light becomes unidirectional and will not be recognized by the detector filter unless it alters its polarity. The polarized light reflected from superficial layers of the skin will remain in its original polarization and thus cannot be detected by the filter. However, polarized light disperses as it goes deeper into the skin and experiences several scattering events resulting in randomization of polarization having most of the light return from the deeper layers [10]. Overall, nonpolarized dermoscopes are better to inspect superficial layers, while polarized dermoscopes are more effective to visualize deeper structures such as vasculature [10]. Interface solutions such as ultrasound gel, antiseptic gel for hands, and alcohol are required for nonpolarized dermoscopes and can be used for polarized dermoscopes [7, 12]. The convexity and hard surface of the nail plate cause liquids to escape easily; as a result, clear viscous ultrasound gel is mostly recommended for better visualization of this area [7, 12]. As for the capillaries of the hyponychium, alcohol is the favored solution as it provides the best image clarity, and the observation can be with a polarized dermoscope [6, 12].

8.4 Clinical Features

Psoriasis can be isolated only to the nail, with diverse manifestations between patients and between the nails of one individual [13]. Depending on the portion of the nail that is affected, dermoscopic features can help diagnose psoriasis and reinforce clinical findings [2, 5]. In particular, dermoscopy allows to better visualize the psoriatic pits and to detect remains of parakeratotic cells inside the depressions with polarized dermoscopy. When examined with a nonpolarized instrument, pits are filled with gel, and dermoscopy shows a peripheral white border (Fig. 8.1). Dermoscopy of onycholysis shows either a homogeneously white area or a white area with multiple thin longitudinal white striae (Fig. 8.2). It also allows seeing the

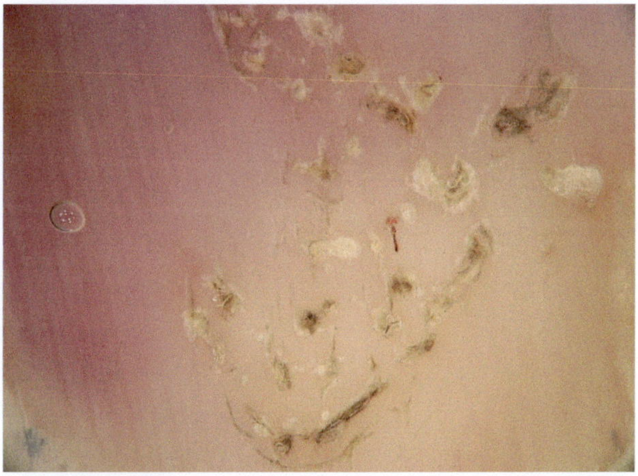

Fig. 8.1 Nail pitting, note presence of scales. Staining is caused by contact with pigmented dyes

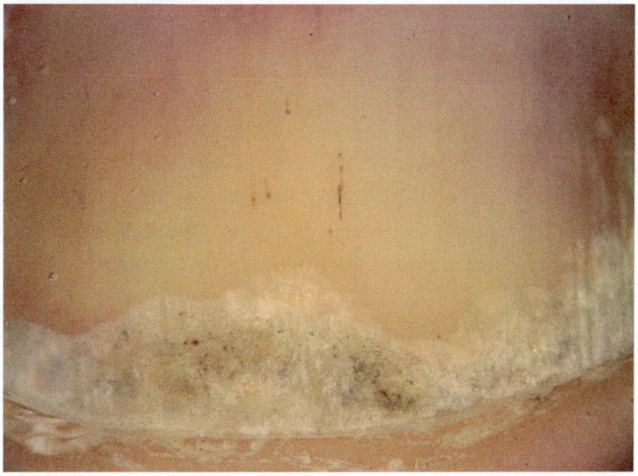

Fig. 8.2 Onycholysis and splinter hemorrhages

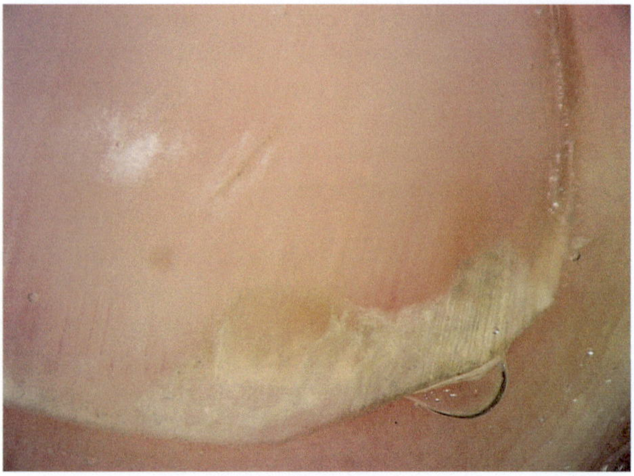

Fig. 8.3 Onycholysis with erythematous border

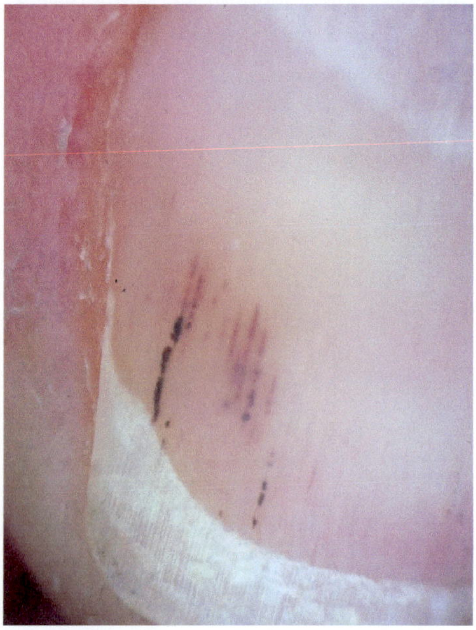

Fig. 8.4 Splinter hemorrhages

erythematous border as a patchy red to orange discoloration of the nail bed surrounding the onycholytic areas, when it is scarcely evident at clinical examination (Fig. 8.3). Splinter hemorrhages can also be very well visualized using dermoscopy; they appear as brown, purple to black spots arranged in a longitudinal fashion (Fig. 8.4). Dilation and tortuosity of the capillary of the distal nail bed is also commonly observed (Fig. 8.5).

Dermoscopy of the hyponychium is very useful as it allows diagnosis of psoriasis in doubtful cases. However it requires a magnification of at least 40× and therefore cannot be performed with a handheld dermoscope but requires the use of a

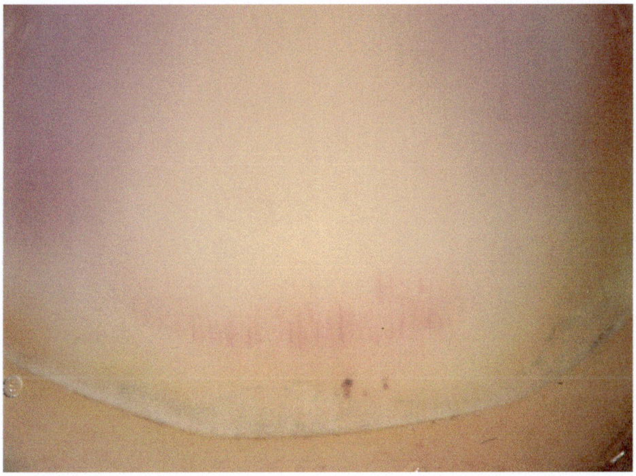

Fig. 8.5 Dilation of distal nail bed capillaries

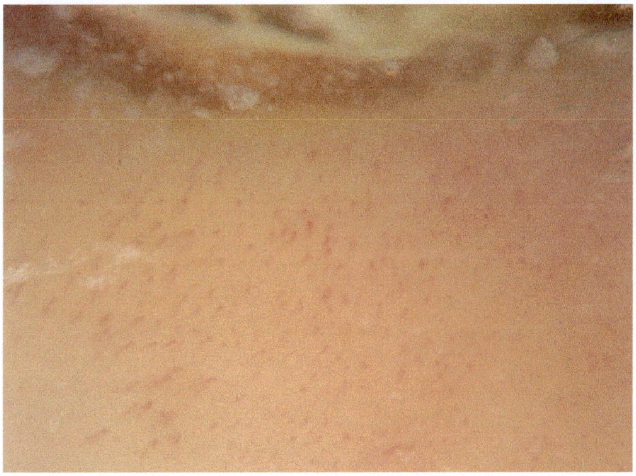

Fig. 8.6 Twisted capillaries at 40× magnification

videodermatoscope. The presence of twisted dilated capillary loops, identical to those observed in the psoriatic scalp, is typical of psoriasis (Figs. 8.6 and 8.7). Dermoscopy of the hyponychium is also useful in the follow-up of nail psoriasis with a positive correlation between reduction in the number of twisted capillaries and response to therapy [6].

Dermoscopy of the proximal nail fold is also useful for assessing the severity of the disease. Studies of dermoscopy of this region have found the number and diameter of capillaries to be significantly decreased in psoriatic patients [14–16]. Another measure of severity of disease is the presence of nail crumbling of the nail plate [7]. With the aid of a dermoscope, the aforementioned features can be better visualized and help the clinician distinguish psoriasis from other nail disorders [8].

Dermoscopic findings of diagnostic features are shown in Table 8.1.

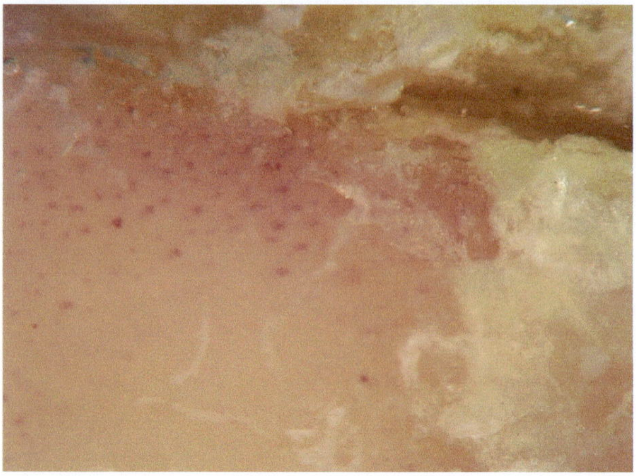

Fig. 8.7 Twisted capillaries, at higher magnification (70×)

Table 8.1 Dermoscopic findings of diagnostic features

Location	Feature	Clinical finding	Dermoscopic description
Nail matrix	Pitting	Large, deep, and irregularly scattered dimples	Concavities that have a white halo and are variable in size and shape
Nail bed	Onycholysis	The nail plate has a white color due to the presence of air between the nail plate and the nail bed. The area is surrounded by an erythematous border	Homogeneous white discoloration or white discoloration with multiple white longitudinal striae surrounded by a yellow to red band
	Salmon patches	Irregular areas of yellowish orange discoloration visible through the nail plate	Areas of yellow to red discoloration that are variable in size and shape
Distal nail bed/hyponychium	Twisted capillary loops		Visible capillaries that look like red dots at low magnification. At 40× magnification, twisted and randomly distributed loops
Proximal nail bed/proximal nail fold	Decreased proximal nail fold capillary density		Decreased number and diameter of capillaries

Summary for Clinician

Dermoscopy is a noninvasive, fast, and relatively straightforward imaging modality that can assist with the diagnosis of nail psoriasis especially in cases of nonspecific nail changes, such as simple onycholysis or isolated subungual hyperkeratosis [6]. Clinicians can also utilize the tool for prognostic evaluation, improving follow-up care and monitoring response to therapy [1]. Dermoscopy represents an indispensible tool that physicians have recently added to their arsenal of approaching and managing onychopathies.

Acknowledgment We want to acknowledge Mrs. Agnese Canazza for her technical support with the images.

References

1. Micali G, Lacarrubba F, Massimino D, Schwartz RA. Dermatoscopy: alternative uses in daily clinical practice. J Am Acad Dermatol. 2011;64(6):1135–46. PubMed PMID: 21292346.
2. Tosti APB, Farias DC. Nail dermoscopy. In: Micali G, editor. Videodermatoscopy in clinical practice. London: Informa Healthcare; 2009.
3. Piraccini BM, Balestri R, Starace M, Rech G. Nail digital dermoscopy (onychoscopy) in the diagnosis of onychomycosis. J Eur Acad Dermatol Venereol. 2013;27(4):509–13. PubMed PMID: 22040510.
4. Nakamura RC, Costa MC. Dermatoscopic findings in the most frequent onychopathies: descriptive analysis of 500 cases. Int J Dermatol. 2012;51(4):483–5. PubMed PMID: 22435443.
5. Farias DC, Tosti A, Chiacchio ND, Hirata SH. [Dermoscopy in nail psoriasis]. An Bras Dermatol. 2010;85(1):101–3. PubMed PMID: 20464097. Aspectos dermatoscopicos na psoriase ungueal.
6. Iorizzo M, Dahdah M, Vincenzi C, Tosti A. Videodermoscopy of the hyponychium in nail bed psoriasis. J Am Acad Dermatol. 2008;58(4):714–5. PubMed PMID: 18342725.
7. Piraccini BM, Bruni F, Starace M. Dermoscopy of non-skin cancer nail disorders. Dermatol Ther. 2012;25(6):594–602. PubMed PMID: 23210758.
8. Lencastre A, Lamas A, Sa D, Tosti A. Onychoscopy. Clin Dermatol. 2013;31(5):587–93. PubMed PMID: 24079588.
9. Argenziano G, Soyer HP. Dermoscopy of pigmented skin lesions – a valuable tool for early diagnosis of melanoma. Lancet Oncol. 2001;2(7):443–9. PubMed PMID: 11905739.
10. Pan Y, Gareau DS, Scope A, Rajadhyaksha M, Mullani NA, Marghoob AA. Polarized and nonpolarized dermoscopy: the explanation for the observed differences. Arch Dermatol. 2008;144(6):828–9. PubMed PMID: 18559791.
11. Benvenuto-Andrade C, Dusza SW, Agero AL, Scope A, Rajadhyaksha M, Halpern AC, et al. Differences between polarized light dermoscopy and immersion contact dermoscopy for the evaluation of skin lesions. Arch Dermatol. 2007;143(3):329–38. PubMed PMID: 17372097.
12. Gewirtzman AJ, Saurat JH, Braun RP. An evaluation of dermoscopy fluids and application techniques. Br J Dermatol. 2003;149(1):59–63. PubMed PMID: 12890195.
13. Tosti A, Daniel R, Piraccini BM, Iorizzo M. Color atlas of nails. Berlin: Springer; 2010.
14. Ohtsuka T, Yamakage A, Miyachi Y. Statistical definition of nail fold capillary pattern in patients with psoriasis. Int J Dermatol. 1994;33(11):779–82. PubMed PMID: 7822081.
15. Zaric D, Clemmensen OJ, Worm AM, Stahl D. Capillary microscopy of the nail fold in patients with psoriasis and psoriatic arthritis. Dermatologica. 1982;164(1):10–4. PubMed PMID: 7067875.
16. Bhushan M, Moore T, Herrick AL, Griffiths CE. Nail fold video capillaroscopy in psoriasis. Br J Dermatol. 2000;142(6):1171–6. PubMed PMID: 10848742.

Severity Evaluation Indexes

9

Dimitrios Rigopoulos and Christos Prevezas

Contents

Key Features

- Severity Evaluation Indexes are very useful tools in daily practice and clinical trials.
- Total NAPSI and Target NAPSI are the most commonly used so far.
- The ideal index would be quick, simple,valid and combine both patient-related and physician-assessed outcome measures.

Severity Evaluation Indexes are very useful instruments for the assessment of a patient with nail psoriasis. Their role is essential in clinical trials, baseline consultation, therapeutic strategy, and consequent follow-up. Therefore, they should be objective, reproducible, and simple to perform.

D. Rigopoulos, MD (✉)
Second Department of Dermatology, Athens University School of Medicine, Athens, Greece
e-mail: drigop@hol.gr

C. Prevezas, MD
Second Department of Dermatology, Attikon University Hospital, Athens, Greece
e-mail: chrisprevezas@yahoo.com

D. Rigopoulos, A. Tosti (eds.), *Nail Psoriasis: From A to Z*,
DOI 10.1007/978-3-319-08810-5_9

Various parameters are taken into account such as localization of the inflammatory process, polymorphism of clinical findings, disease extent, and quality of life impairment. In order to assess disease severity, studies have either focused on one specific clinical sign [1, 2] or have tried to combine multiple features to improve their validity. Qualitative assessment is quicker but, on the other hand, grades subjectively the severity of each feature. Numeric or quantitative evaluation is more objective but is more time-consuming.

9.1 NAPSI (Nail Psoriasis Severity Index)

9.1.1 Total NAPSI

Rich and Scher [3] published in 2003 a numeric, reproducible, and objective index named Nail Psoriasis Severity Index (NAPSI). This index has been widely used so far in clinical trials [4–8] and daily practice.

The nail is divided into quadrants with imaginary horizontal and longitudinal lines. Then, each quadrant is evaluated for the presence or absence of any of the features of *nail matrix* (pitting, leukonychia, red spots in the lunula, nail plate crumbling) and *nail bed* (onycholysis, oil-drop dyschromia, subungual hyperkeratosis) psoriasis (Table 9.1). Findings of psoriatic arthritis (PsoA) or pustular psoriasis are not taken into consideration. Psoriasis of the proximal nail fold is excluded as well and should be assessed with concomitant cutaneous lesions. The absence of any nail bed and matrix psoriasis in a quadrant has a score of zero. The score is one if features are present in one quarter, two if present in two quarters, three if present in three quarters, and four if present in four quarters. If more than one feature of the same category (matrix or bed psoriasis) is present in the same quarter of the nail, the score remains, nevertheless, unchangeable. For example, while the presence of pits in one quadrant has a score of 1, the score is similar if pits and any other matrix feature coexist in the same quadrant. The highest score possible for each fingernail is 8 (4 for bed plus 4 for matrix psoriasis) for a total of 80 for all fingernails. If toenails are included, then the maximum total number increases to 160 (Table 9.2). Although original NAPSI was rated only on fingernails, it is been shown that it can be applied

Table 9.1 NAPSI clinical features

Nail matrix psoriasis	Nail bed psoriasis
Pitting	Onycholysis
Leukonychia	Oil drop (salmon patch)
Red spots in the lunula	Splinter hemorrhages
Nail plate crumbling	Subungual hyperkeratosis

Table 9.2 NAPSI scoring

Scoring each quadrant	Total score
0 = absence of findings	Single nail = 0–8
1 = present in 1/4 (nail)	All fingernails = 0–80
2 = present in 2/4 nail	All toenails = 0–80
3 = present in 3/4 nail	Total NAPSI score = 0–160
4 = present in 4/4 nail	

on toenails as well [9]. It should also be noted that the authors conducted a real-time assessment of patients and did not review any photographic material of their patients.

9.1.2 Target NAPSI

As an alternative to the total NAPSI score, the term *target nail* was introduced corresponding to the most severely affected nail among all at baseline. This time, every feature is graded with a maximum score of 8 per quadrant and 32 for the whole nail. The target nail remains the same nail throughout the study, even if that nail is no longer the most affected.

Parrish et al. [10] published a modification of target NAPSI based on the fact that each feature is graded depending on its presence or absence rather than its severity. They proposed a qualitative assessment from 0 to 3 (0 = none, 1 = mild, 2 = moderate, and 3 = severe), to be added for each parameter of target NAPSI. This modification augments the overall scoring from 32 to 96 rendering the index more precise but on the other hand more copious to perform in clinical practice.

Target NAPSI is probably less representative than the total NAPSI when assessing treatment response [11] and should be combined with other indexes (e.g., Nail Physician Global Assessment – Nail PGA) when used in clinical trials.

9.1.3 NAPSI Reconsidered

Several studies [12–14] have questioned the content of NAPSI regarding the presence or absence of clinical features. Van der Velden et al. [12] concluded that all features of NAPSI are frequent in psoriatic patients except leukonychia. The latter feature did not show a higher prevalence comparing with the control group. Therefore, the authors propose this feature not be included in a nail psoriasis index tool. Garzitto et al. [13] found similar results in a study with a higher number of patients. Moreover other features not included in NAPSI, such as longitudinal ridges, nail fold involvement, longitudinal ridges, and Beau's lines/onychomadesis, showed a significantly higher prevalence in psoriatic patients compared with control subjects.

Aktan et al. [9] rated the interobserver reliability of the NAPSI score and found it to be better for nail bed rather than matrix features. Difficulties during evaluation of small toenail surfaces and the exclusion of features such as the longitudinal ridges and Beau's lines can end up with this difference. In the same study, pitting, oil-drop dyschromia, and subungual hyperkeratosis were the most common features, while leukonychia was the less frequent.

9.1.4 Modified NAPSI

In an effort to improve NAPSI, Cassell et al. published the *modified NAPSI* [8], a simpler and more practical version, that showed good inter- and intrarater reliability. Fingernails are no longer divided into quadrants. The features to be evaluated

Table 9.3 Modified NAPSI

Score	Pits (number of)	Nail plate crumbling	Onycholysis and/or oil-drop dyschromia[a]
0	None	Absent	Absent
1	1–10	1–25 % of the nail	1–10 % of the nail
2	11–49	26–50 % of the nail	11–30 % of the nail
3	≥50	>50 % of the nail	>30 % of the nail
		Red spots in the lunula	
0 if absent		**Nail bed hyperkeratosis**	
1 if present		**Leukonychia**	
		Splinter hemorrhages	

[a]Onycholysis and oil-drop dyschromia are evaluated together

are now seven instead of eight used for the NAPSI. Pitting, onycholysis and oil-drop dyschromia, and nail plate crumbling are graded from 0 to 3 in severity. Leukonychia, splinter hemorrhages, hyperkeratosis, and red spots in the lunula are graded as either present or absent (Table 9.3). The score ranges from 0 to 13 for each fingernail and 0–130 for all fingernails.

The modified NAPSI has been a work of rheumatologists with dermatologist's input. The study has assessed patients with nail psoriasis and psoriatic arthritis (PsA) so as to create a simpler tool to be used in clinical trials. Comparing to NAPSI, patient evaluation was based on photographic material. Seven (instead of eight in NAPSI) features are to be evaluated as onycholysis is merged with salmon patch dyschromia and are assessed together. Patients were suffering from psoriatic arthritis and were, in majority, actively treated with DMARDs (disease modifying antirheumatic drugs) and/or biologic agents. During this study, the modified NAPSI was compared with other psoriasis and psoriatic arthritis indexes for a better understanding of correlations.

Physician global PsA disease severity and physician nail severity VAS (visual analog scale) correlated significantly. On the contrary, modified NAPSI did not correlate with PASI, global skin and nail disease severity VAS scores, patient global arthritis and skin severity VAS scores, and HAQ (Health Assessment Questionnaire) scores.

9.2 NAPPA (Nail Assessment in Psoriasis and Psoriatic Arthritis)

Recently, a multicenter effort has led to the development of a new assessment tool called NAPPA [15]. It is divided in three parts:

(a) *NAPPA-QoL* (*quality of life*) is a questionnaire that assesses patient's quality of life. Questions focus on the intensity of complaints during the last week and are rated on a 5-option scale (scored 0–4).
(b) *NAPPA-PBI* (*patient benefit index*) is also a patient questionnaire comprised of two parts. The first part is answered before treatment initiation. It is called PNQ

Table 9.4 BARAN's index

Score	Pits (number of)	Beau's lines	Subungual hyperkeratosis[a] (mm)	Onycholysis[b] (%)
1 (slight)	<10	1 groove	<2	<25
2 (moderate)	10–20	2–3 grooves	2–3	25–50
3 (severe)	>20	>3 grooves	>3	>50

[a]Subungual hyperkeratosis is measured with a caliper
[b]Onycholysis, trachyonychia, leukonychia, and oily spots are graded separately in the same manner. The nail is divided into eight equal portions (each portion accounts for 12.5 % of the whole nail)

or Patient Needs Questionnaire and rates the importance of 24 treatment goals on a 5-option scale. The second part is answered during or after therapy. It is a questionnaire similar to PNQ where the extent of satisfaction of each treatment goal is evaluated.

(c) *NAPPA-CLIN* (*clinical*) is a brief version of NAPSI that assesses only four digits instead of 20 digits (the sum of the least and worst affected among all toenails and fingernails). It was found to correlate highly with the total NAPSI score.

NAPPA is a quick, valid, feasible, and reliable instrument that combines patient's overview on the disease as well as physician's perspective. It remains to be used in clinical trials for further evaluation.

9.3 Baran's Nail Psoriasis Severity Index

Baran [16] devised a numeric system that categorizes clinical features according to the site of the pathology. The clinician grades the severity of each clinical sign and sums up for the final score (Table 9.4). Nail signs can originate from the *proximal matrix* (pits, Beau's lines, onychomadesis and nail loss, trachyonychia), *intermediate matrix* (leukonychia), *subungual tissues distal to the lunula* (hyperkeratosis, onycholysis, splinter hemorrhages, oil spots), or involve the whole nail unit.

However, splinter hemorrhages are thought to be traumatic and excluded from grading. Onychomadesis and nail loss are not taken into account as well.

9.4 Cannavò's Scoring System

During a study for the assessment of a topical solution with cyclosporin, Cannavò et al. [17] evaluated five clinical signs of fingernail psoriasis (onycholysis, pitting, hyperkeratosis, nail plate crumbling, oil-drop dyschromia) before and after the treatment. The severity of each feature was graded from 0 (absent) to 3 (severe). Additionally, patients were asked to assess their disease severity, life impairment, and the treatment's efficacy. Cannavò's scoring system is a qualitative, quick, and practical system. Nevertheless, its inter-rater reliability has not been established.

9.5 Nail PGA (Nail Physician's Global Assessment)

Similar to PGA, the physician assesses quickly the severity of the disease with a 4- or 5-point scale (1 = none, 2 = mild, 3 = moderate, 4 = severe, and 5 = very severe). It is a subjective index used as an adjuvant and not as a stand-alone tool [18].

9.6 NPQ10 (Nail Psoriasis Quality of Life Scale)

Ortonne et al. [19] developed a ten-item questionnaire that evaluates the impact of nail psoriasis on the patient's functional status and quality of life. The study included a large random sample of 4,000 patients. Female gender, a shorter psoriasis history, and dual location were all associated with significantly higher NPQ10 scores, indicating greater impairment. Comparison of NPQ10 with DLQI showed good agreement. The scale has not been tested yet in longitudinal studies.

Conclusion

There is a need for accurate and valid evaluation of nail psoriatic disease. Many authors have tried to implement instruments used either in clinical trials or during the evaluation of various treatments. A recent retrospective study of assessment tools for nail psoriasis found total NAPSI and target NAPSI to be the most commonly used indexes so far [20] in clinical trials. Still these indexes have their limitations as mentioned above and do not include nail psoriasis' impact on health-related quality of life. The optimal nail psoriasis index would be quick, simple, and valid and would include both patient-related and physician-assessed outcomes measures.

References

1. Tosti A, Piraccini BM, Cameli N, Kokely F, Plozzer C, Cannata GE, et al. Calcipotriol ointment in nail psoriasis: a controlled double-blind comparison with betamethasone dipropionate and salicylic acid. Br J Dermatol. 1998;139:655–9.
2. Pierard GE, Pierard-Franchmimont C. Dynamics of psoriatic trachyonychia during low-dose cyclosporin A treatment: a pilot study on onychochronobiology using optical profilometry. Dermatology. 1996;192:116–9.
3. Rich P, Scher R. Nail psoriasis severity index: a useful tool for evaluation of nail psoriasis. J Am Acad Dermatol. 2003;49:206–12.
4. Rigopoulos D, Gregoriou S, Makris M, et al. Efficacy of Ustekinumab in nail psoriasis and improvement in nail-associated quality of life in a population treated with Ustekinumab for cutaneous psoriasis: an open prospective unblinded study. Dermatology. 2011;223(4):325–9.
5. Tosti A, Ricotti C, Romanelli P, et al. Evaluation of the efficacy of Acitretin therapy for nail psoriasis. Arch Dermatol. 2009;145(3):269–71.
6. Bianchi L, Bergamin A, de Felice C, et al. Remission and time of resolution of nail psoriasis during Infliximab therapy. J Am Acad Dermatol. 2005;52(4):736–7.

7. Bardazzi F, Antonucci VA, Tengattini V, et al. A 36-week retrospective open trial comparing the efficacy of biological therapies in nail psoriasis. J Dtsch Dermatol Ges. 2013;11(11): 1065–70.
8. Cassell SE et al. The modified Nail Psoriasis Severity Index: validation of an instrument to assess psoriatic nail involvement in patients with psoriatic arthritis. J Rheumatol. 2007;34: 123–9.
9. Aktan S, Ilknur T, Akin C, et al. Interobserver reliability of the Nail Psoriasis Severity Index. Clin Exp Dermatol. 2007;32:141–4.
10. Parrish CA, Sobera JO, Elewski BO. Modification of Nail Psoriasis Severity Index. J Am Acad Dermatol. 2005;53(4):745–6; author reply 746–7.
11. Rich P, Scher R. Modifications of the Nail Psoriasis Severity Index [authors reply]. J Am Acad Dermatol. 2005;53:746–7.
12. van der Velden HM, Klaassen KM, van de Kerkhof PC, et al. Fingernail psoriasis reconsidered: a case-control study. J Am Acad Dermatol. 2013;69:245–52.
13. Garzitto A, Ricceri R, Trip L, et al. Possible reconsideration of the Nail Psoriasis Severity Index (NAPSI) score. J Am Acad Dermatol. 2013;69(6):1053–4.
14. Kacar N, Ergin S, Erdogan B. The comparison of Nail Psoriasis Severity Index with a less time-consuming qualitative system. J Eur Acad Dermatol Venereol. 2008;22:219–22.
15. Augustin M, Blome C, Costanzo A, et al. Nail Assessment in Psoriasis and Psoriatic Arthritis (NAPPA): development and validation of a tool for assessment of nail psoriasis outcomes. Br J Dermatol. 2014;170(3):591–8.
16. Baran RL. A nail psoriasis severity index. Br J Dermatol. 2004;150:568–9.
17. Cannavò SP, Guarneri F, Vaccaro M, et al. Treatment of psoriatic nails with topical cyclosporin: a prospective, randomized placebo-controlled study. Dermatology. 2003;206:153–6.
18. Rich P, Bourcier M, Sofen H, et al. The PHOENIX 1 Investigators. Ustekinumab improves nail disease in patients with moderate-to-severe psoriasis: results from PHOENIX 1. Br J Dermatol. 2014;170(2):398–407.
19. Ortonne JP, Baran R, Corvest M, et al. Development and validation of nail psoriasis quality of life scale (NPQ10). J Eur Acad Dermatol Venereol. 2010;24:22–7.
20. Augustin M, Ogilvie A. Methods of outcomes measurement in nail psoriasis. Dermatology. 2010;221 Suppl 1:23–8.

Quality of Life

10

Stamatis Gregoriou and Dimitris Rigopoulos

Contents

Key Features

- Nail psoriasis results in significant impairment to health-related quality of life (HRQOL). Specific nail psoriasis questionnaires have been developed to evaluate the impact of nail psoriasis on HRQOL.
- Improvement of nail psoriasis through treatment results in significant improvement of HRQOL.

Nail psoriasis causes significant impairment in health-related quality of life (HRQOL) affecting physical activities as well as emotional status and social behavior of patients. De Jong reported that 93 % of the patients consider nail psoriasis a major cosmetic issue, 52 % experience pain in daily activities, and 48 % report associated problems in their occupation [1]. Nail involvement in psoriasis has been associated with a significantly greater area of the skin affected [2], longer duration of the disease [3], as well as higher prevalence of psoriatic arthritis [4] adding to the

S. Gregoriou, MD, PhD
Second Department of Dermatology, University of Athens Medical School, Attikon Hospital, Athens, Greece
e-mail: stamgreg@yahoo.gr

D. Rigopoulos, MD (✉)
Second Department of Dermatology, Athens University School of Medicine, Athens, Greece
e-mail: drigop@hol.gr

D. Rigopoulos, A. Tosti (eds.), *Nail Psoriasis: From A to Z*,
DOI 10.1007/978-3-319-08810-5_10

burden of HRQOL. Among patients with psoriatic arthritis, nail involvement has been associated with higher anxiety and depression scores [1]. The impact of nail psoriasis on HRQOL has been evaluated through classic instruments such as DLQI as well as disease-specific indexes.

10.1 Burden of Nail Psoriasis as Estimated by HRQOL Indexes

Classic questionnaires allow comparison of impact of nail psoriasis on HRQOL with other dermatological disorders. Patients with nail psoriasis display a significantly lower quality of life in the DLQI and a poorer state of health in general HRQOL instruments such as the Euroqol (EQ5-D) when compared to patients with just skin psoriasis [2]. They also report significantly worse values for satisfaction with their treatment, stress, and time expenditure due to therapy. The mean number of consultations is significantly higher in nail psoriasis patients, both with dermatologists and with orthopedic surgeons/rheumatologists [2]. Nail psoriasis also results in significantly more days off from work [5].

Specific nail psoriasis questionnaires are more accurate at evaluating the impairment caused by just nail involvement without additional confounding factors. Ortonne et al. used both DLQI and a newly designed nail-specific tool (the NPQ10 questionnaire) to evaluate quality of life in patients with nail psoriasis [6]. Even though only 1,309 questionnaires were returned out of 4,000 sent, the authors showed a good agreement between DLQI and NPQ10 tools. Patients reported nail psoriasis to be bothersome (86 %), unsightly (87 %), and painful (59 %) with significant lower QoL. A study comparing the burden on HRQOL between different nail disorders concluded that patients in the population studied experienced similar impairment in their QoL by psoriasis, onychomycosis, chromonychia, and even trauma. Burden on both physical and emotional components in this population was associated with the number of nails affected, but not with a particular nail disorder [7].

10.2 Effect of Nail Psoriasis Therapy on HRQOL

Expert opinion suggests that treatment options of psoriasis in this era should be selected and modified based on whether treatment goals are met or failed. A recent consensus reported that "there is no generally accepted consensus definition of either treatment success or failure and a lack of a definition of a sufficient improvement in an individual patient's disease, but it likely depends on a combination of the drug's effectiveness, convenience and safety and patient-reported outcomes such as preference, satisfaction and improvement in HRQOL" [8]. The European S3-guidelines on the systemic treatment of psoriasis in 2009 propose 75 % or more improvement in the Psoriasis Area and Severity Index from baseline (PASI 75) and a Dermatology Life Quality Index (DLQI) of 0 or 1 as treatment goals [9]. However, studies demonstrate that such a goal is difficult to achieve since a PASI 90 response may be necessary to achieve a DLQI of 0 or 1 [10]. There are no index-based treatment goals for nail psoriasis. There are no data in medical literature evaluating the improvement of HRQOL in patients using topical treatment for nail psoriasis, but data suggest that treatment should be maintained for months and a 90 % improvement in nail area and severity index (NAPSI) is difficult to achieve. Systemic treatment of nail psoriasis results in significant improvement both in NAPSI and HRQOL particularly in patients treated with biologics [11–13]. However, there is still controversy among experts regarding the use of biologics in patients with nail psoriasis without extensive cutaneous or joint involvement.

In present day health economics settings, the challenge posed is to strive for a balance between cost-effectiveness and evaluating HRQOL when making therapeutic choices, particularly in diseases with prolonged duration such as nail psoriasis.

References

1. de Jong EM, Seegers BA, Gulinck MK, et al. Psoriasis of the nails associated with disability in a large number of patients: results of a recent interview with 1,728 patients. Dermatology. 1996;193:300–3.
2. Radtke MA, Langenbruch AK, Schäfer I, Herberger K, Reich K, Augustin M. Nail psoriasis as a severity indicator: results from the PsoReal study. Patient Relat Outcome Meas. 2011;2:1–6.
3. Feldman SR, Fleischer Jr AB, Reboussin DM, Rapp SR, Bradham DD, Exum ML, Clark AR. The economic impact of psoriasis increases with psoriasis severity. J Am Acad Dermatol. 1997;37:564–9.
4. Wilson FC, Icen M, Crowson CS, McEvoy MT, Gabriel SE, Kremers HM. Incidence and clinical predictors of psoriatic arthritis in patients with psoriasis: a population-based study. Arthritis Rheum. 2009;61:233–9. doi:10.1002/art.24172.
5. Augustin M, Reich K, Blome C, et al. Nail psoriasis in Germany: epidemiology and burden of disease. Br J Dermatol. 2010;163:580–5.
6. Ortonne JP, Baran R, Corvest M, et al. Development and validation of nail psoriasis quality of life scale (NPQ10). J Eur Acad Dermatol Venereol. 2010;24:22–7.
7. Belyayeva E, Gregoriou S, Chalikias J, Kontochristopoulos G, Koumantaki E, Makris M, Koti I, Katoulis A, Katsambas A, Rigopoulos D. The impact of nail disorders on quality of life. Eur J Dermatol. 2013;23(3):366–71.
8. Mrowietz U, Kragballe K, Reich K, Spuls P, Griffiths CE, Nast A, Franke J, Antoniou C, Arenberger P, Balieva F, Bylaite M, Correia O, Daudén E, Gisondi P, Iversen L, Kemény L, Lahfa M, Nijsten T, Rantanen T, Reich A, Rosenbach T, Segaert S, Smith C, Talme T, Volc-Platzer B, Yawalkar N. Definition of treatment goals for moderate to severe psoriasis: a European consensus. Arch Dermatol Res. 2011;303:1–10.
9. Pathirana D, Ormerod AD, Saiag P, Smith C, Spuls PI, Nast A, Barker J, Bos JD, Burmester GR, Chimenti S, Dubertret L, Eberlein B, Erdmann R, Ferguson J, Girolomoni G, Gisondi P, Giunta A, Griffiths C, Hönigsmann H, Hussain M, Jobling R, Karvonen SL, Kemeny L, Kopp I, Leonardi C, Maccarone M, Menter A, Mrowietz U, Naldi L, Nijsten T, Ortonne JP, Orzechowski HD, Rantanen T, Reich K, Reytan N, Richards H, Thio HB, van de Kerkhof P, Rzany B. European S3-guidelines on the systemic treatment of psoriasis vulgaris. J Eur Acad Dermatol Venereol. 2009;23 Suppl 2:1–70. doi:10.1111/j.1468-3083.2009.03389.x. Erratum in: J Eur Acad Dermatol Venereol. 2010;24(1):117–8.
10. Torii H, Sato N, Yoshinari T, Nakagawa H, Japanese Infliximab Study Investigators. Dramatic impact of a Psoriasis Area and Severity Index 90 response on the quality of life in patients with psoriasis: an analysis of Japanese clinical trials of infliximab. J Dermatol. 2012;39(3):253–9.

11. Rigopoulos D, Gregoriou S, Stratigos A, et al. Evaluation of the efficacy and safety of infliximab on psoriatic nails: an unblinded, nonrandomized, open-label study. Br J Dermatol. 2008;159:453–6.
12. Rigopoulos D, Gregoriou S, Lazaridou E, et al. Treatment of nail psoriasis with adalimumab: an open label unblinded study. J Eur Acad Dermatol Venereol. 2010;24:530–4.
13. Rigopoulos D, Gregoriou S, Makris M, Ioannides D. Efficacy of ustekinumab in nail psoriasis and improvement in nail-associated quality of life in a population treated with ustekinumab for cutaneous psoriasis: an open prospective unblinded study. Dermatology. 2011;223:325–9.

Differential Diagnosis for Nail Psoriasis

11

Natalie C. Yin and Antonella Tosti

Contents

Key Features

- Several diseases can cause nail abnormalities similar to those in nail psoriasis. The most important differential diagnoses include alopecia areata, idiopathic onycholysis, and traumatic nail disorders.
- A diagnosis of onychomycosis does not exclude nail psoriasis as the two conditions are commonly associated.
- A good history is invaluable in determining the correct diagnosis.
- Exam of all 20 nails is always necessary.

N.C. Yin, BS (✉)
Department of Dermatology and Cutaneous Surgery,
University of Miami, Miami, FL, USA
e-mail: nyin@med.miami.edu

A. Tosti, MD (✉)
Department of Dermatology and Cutaneous Surgery, University of Miami
Miller School of Medicine, Miami, FL, USA
e-mail: antonella.tosti@unibo.it

D. Rigopoulos, A. Tosti (eds.), *Nail Psoriasis: From A to Z*,
DOI 10.1007/978-3-319-08810-5_11

11.1 Introduction

Nail involvement occurs in up to 50 % of patients with psoriasis [1]. Although most patients experience concurrent skin involvement, 1–5 % of patients present with nail changes alone [2]. In these patients, it can be diagnostically challenging, as psoriatic nail disease can resemble several other nail dystrophies.

In this chapter, we describe the differential diagnoses for each classic sign of nail psoriasis including pitting, onycholysis, subungual hyperkeratosis, splinter hemorrhages, and oil spots [3].

11.2 Nail Plate Pitting

Common causes of nail pitting include psoriasis, alopecia areata, and eczema. A few pits can also be seen in normal nails. Uncommon causes include parakeratosis pustulosa, pemphigus vulgaris, sarcoidosis, dermatomyositis, drug-induced erythroderma, secondary syphilis, Reiter's disease, chronic renal failure/hemodialysis, and chronic paronychia [4] (Table 11.1).

Certain characteristics of nail pitting can help to identify its etiology (Table 11.2). Psoriatic pits are typically deep, indicating involvement of the intermediate and ventral nail plate [5]. Moreover, presence of more than 20 pits is suggestive of psoriatic nail disease [6]. Over 60 pits has been said to be diagnostic of psoriasis [7]. In contrast, pits in alopecia areata are small, superficial and usually arranged in a regularly distributed geometric pattern [8] (Fig. 11.1). They may demonstrate a "rippled" effect [9] and run along longitudinal or transverse lines [8]. Other nail signs of alopecia areata include mottled erythema of the lunula, onychomadesis, and trachyonychia [6, 10]. Pits in eczema are coarse, very irregular and associated with cross ridging [8] The term elkonyxis describes a very large irregular depression, which can be seen in syphilis, Reiter's disease, following a traumatic event, or after isotretinoin therapy [6, 11]. Small pitted craters on the middle and ring fingers, known as Rosenaus depressions, are characteristically seen in patients with diabetes mellitus [12]. It is important to remember that an isolated pit is not diagnostic and may be idiopathic in nature [9].

Table 11.1 Causes of nail pitting [4, 9]

Nail pitting	
Common causes	Uncommon causes
Psoriasis	Normal
Alopecia areata	Parakeratosis pustulosa
Eczema	Pityriasis rosea
Trauma	Hemodialysis
	Chronic renal failure
	Pemphigus vulgaris
	Sarcoidosis
	Dermatomyositis
	Drug-induced erythroderma
	Secondary syphilis

Table 11.2 Differential diagnosis for nail pitting

Pitting	
Cause	Pitting type
Psoriasis	Deep involving intermediate and ventral nail plate
	>20 pits
Alopecia areata	Small, superficial pits
	Regularly distributed, in geometric pattern
	"Rippled" effect, along longitudinal or transverse lines
	Also associated with punctate leukonychia, onychomadesis, or trachyonychia
Eczema	Coarse, irregular pitting, and cross ridging
Syphilis, Reiter's disease, trauma, isotretinoin therapy	Elkonyxis (very large pits)
Diabetes mellitus	Rosenaus depressions – small pits on middle and ring fingers
Idiopathic	Isolated pit

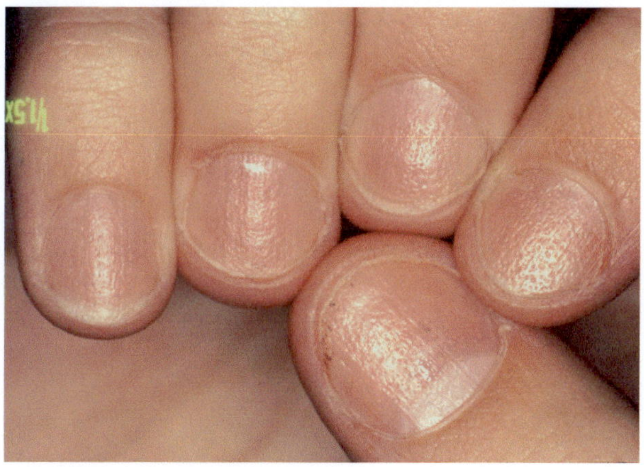

Fig. 11.1 Pitting in alopecia areata

11.3 Onycholysis

The differential diagnosis for onycholysis depends on its location (Table 11.3). The most common cause of onycholysis in fingernails is idiopathic onycholysis (Fig. 11.2). More common in women, idiopathic onycholysis has been speculated to arise secondary to the same environmental factors that result in chronic paronychia [4]. Frequent wetting, irritant contact, or aggressive manicure can damage the onychocorneal band, resulting in nail plate detachment [13]. The onycholytic space is frequently colonized by bacteria and yeast, including *Pseudomonas*, causing a typical green discoloration (Fig. 11.3). Irregularly sculpted onycholysis ("rollercoaster onycholysis") may be an indication of overzealous manicuring [9] and is often associated with striate leukonychia [14] (Fig. 11.4). Occupational onycholysis is seen in hairdressers and butchers.

Table 11.3 Causes of onycholysis [8, 9, 16]

Onycholysis	
Common causes	Uncommon causes
Manicuring ("rollercoaster onycholysis")	Photo-onycholysis
Idiopathic	Bullous disease
Psoriasis	Lichen planus
Onychomycosis	Lichen striatus
Drugs	Connective tissue disorders
Contact dermatitis	Metabolic disorders (e.g., thyrotoxicosis)
Subungual tumors (1 digit)	

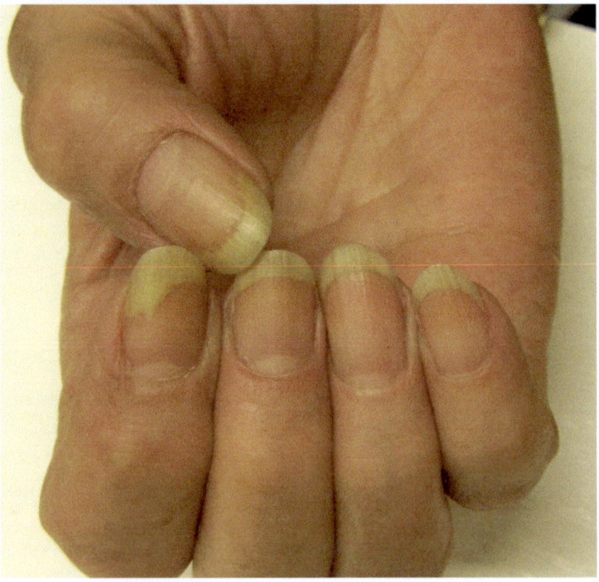

Fig. 11.2 Idiopathic onycholysis

Psoriatic nail onycholysis may be distinguished by the presence of an erythematous rim surrounding the area of onycholysis [3], a finding almost exclusively seen in the fingernails. Moreover, Dawber et al. found that the rate of growth of normal fingernails can help discriminate psoriatic nail versus idiopathic onycholysis. While they described a faster growth rate in nails affected by both psoriatic and idiopathic onycholysis, they found a slightly slower than normal growth rate in the normal nails of idiopathic onycholysis as compared to the normal nails in psoriasis [15].

Other dermatologic conditions causing onycholysis, with a predilection for the fingernails, include eczematous dermatitis and lichen planus. In lichen planus, onycholysis is usually associated with onychorrhexis and other signs of nail matrix involvement (Fig. 11.5). Pompholyx can cause very distal onycholysis affecting most digits [14].

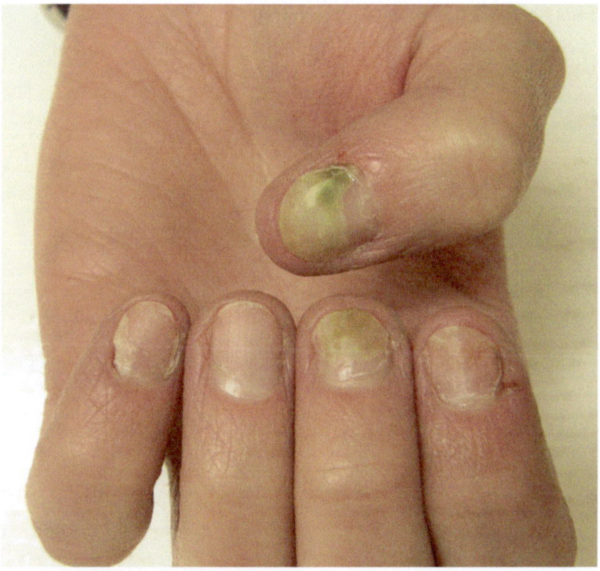

Fig. 11.3 Idiopathic onycholysis featuring green subungual discoloration secondary to pseudomonal infection

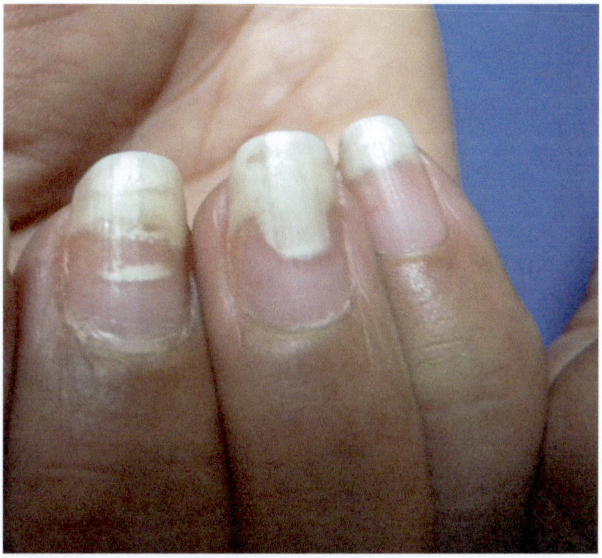

Fig. 11.4 Onycholysis and leukonychia due to manicuring

The two main causes of onycholysis in the toenails are trauma and onychomycosis [9]. Toe stubbing and ill-fitting shoes can lead to nail plate detachment [14]. Onycholysis of the great toe due to an overriding second toe is common and involves the lateral side of the nail [9] (Fig. 11.6). The presence of hemorrhage is a clue for a traumatic cause [16].

Differentiating distal subungual onychomycosis from psoriasis is especially challenging in the toenails. Onychomycosis can be distinguished by the presence of

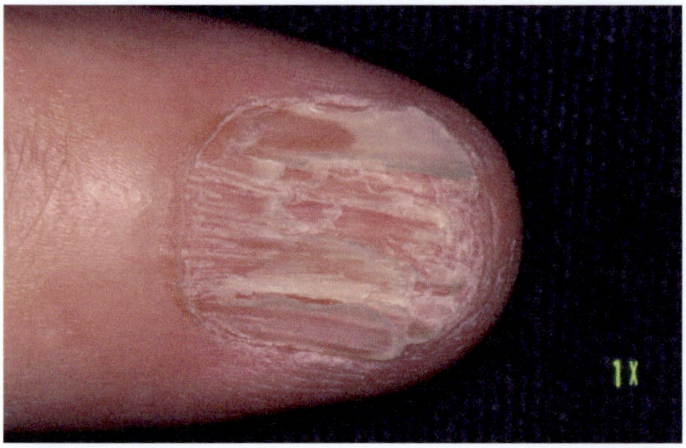

Fig. 11.5 Lichen planus: onycholysis and onychorrhexis

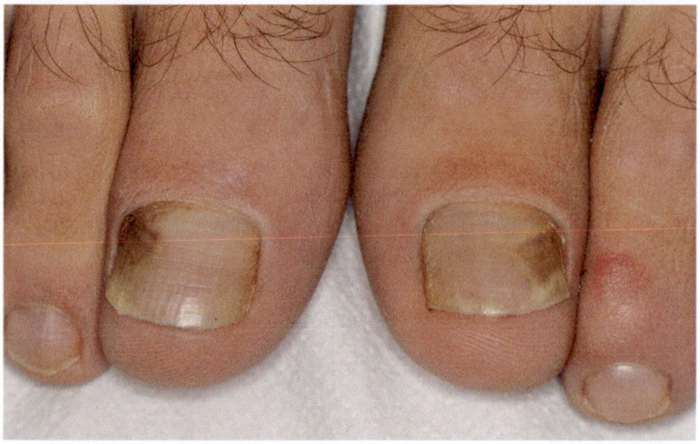

Fig. 11.6 Great toe onycholysis due to overlapping second toe

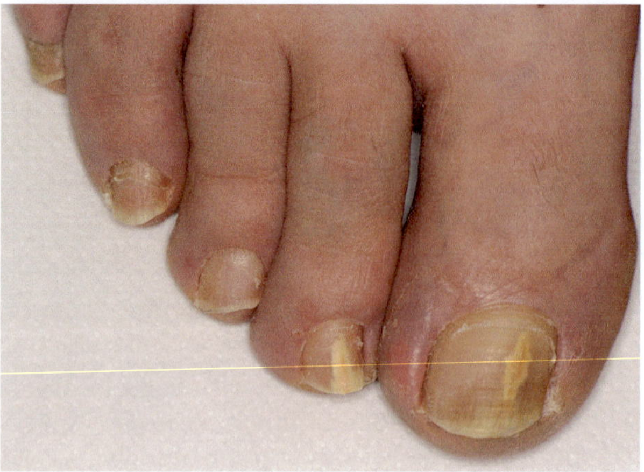

Fig. 11.7 Onychomycosis with yellow patches and strikes

other nail findings, particularly yellow patches and strikes (Fig. 11.7). It is important to consider the possible coexistence of both diseases, which was reported to occur in 48 % of patients [3, 17]. The concomitant conditions are thought to

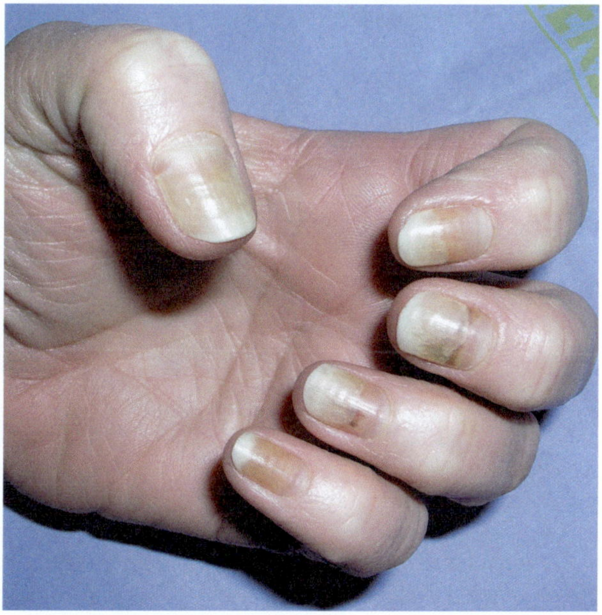

Fig. 11.8 Hemorrhagic onycholysis from taxane use

exacerbate each other, as well. While nail psoriasis itself has been deemed a risk factor for developing onychomycosis [18], Kacar et al. observed more severe nail changes in patients with onychomycosis and suggested the possibility of worsening nail psoriasis by fungal infection via Koebnerization [19]. Ultimately, a fungal and/or bacterial culture in addition to nail plate PAS should be obtained to rule out an infectious etiology [16].

Another cause of toenail onycholysis includes congenital malalignment of the big toenail in children [9].

Drugs can cause onycholysis and less frequently photo-onycholysis. Painful hemorrhagic onycholysis is a common side effect of treatment with taxanes, particularly docetaxel (Fig. 11.8). It is associated with subungual abscesses and usually involves several or all nails. The pathogenesis may be due to direct nail bed toxicity or disruption of nail bed angiogenesis. This complication can increase the risk of sepsis and may require treatment interruption [20].

Photo-onycholysis is rare and most commonly seen with psoralens and tetracycline use [16]. The onycholytic area demonstrates a characteristic hemorrhagic hue [14]. Most nails are affected but the thumbs are usually spared. There are four different subtypes of drug-induced photo-onycholysis: (1) the separation of the nail plate affects several nails and is concave distally with well-demarcated pigmentation proximally, (2) involving a single digit – well-demarcated, circular notch with the widest part distally and brownish pigmentation proximally, (3) round yellow staining (and later reddish) in the center of the nail bed with no lateral or distal margin involvement and affecting several digits, and (4) subungual bullae reported secondary to tetracycline hydrochloride use [9, 21].

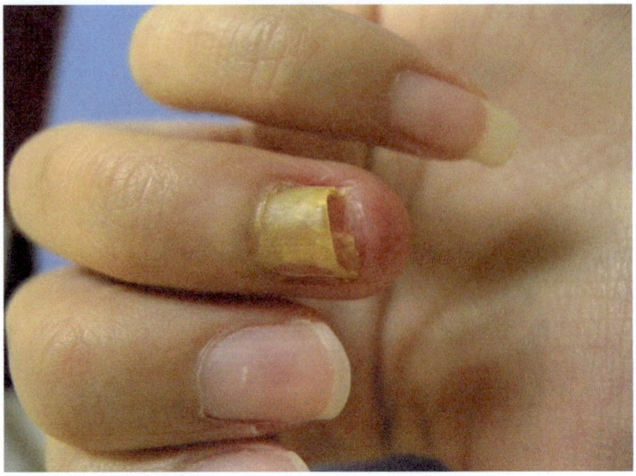

Fig. 11.9 Subungual tumor

Tetracycline or psoralen-induced photo-onycholysis can be painful [4]. Photo-onycholysis may also be observed as part of Segal's triad – photosensitivity, onycholysis, and nail dyschromia [9, 22].

Metabolic disorders, particularly hyperthyroidism, have been reported to cause onycholysis. Plummer nail, a type of onycholysis in which the distal end of the nail curves upward and is undulated, is characteristic of thyrotoxicosis [23].

Onycholysis limited to one nail requires the exclusion of a subungual tumor as the cause. Tumors that can cause onycholysis include subungual exostoses, subungual fibromas, squamous cell carcinomas, and even melanoma [14] (Fig. 11.9). Radiography and/or biopsy is important for diagnosis [16].

Other uncommon causes of onycholysis include lichen striatus, sarcoidosis, and blistering diseases [16, 24].

11.4 Subungual Hyperkeratosis

Subungual hyperkeratosis is most commonly found in nail psoriasis or onychomycosis, although it may also be seen in eczema (Fig. 11.10), lichen planus, pityriasis rubra pilaris, and even cutaneous T cell lymphomas [9, 16]. Usually subungual hyperkeratosis is found in conjunction with onycholysis [9]. The nail bed hyperkeratosis seen in psoriasis is usually silvery white in colour. In onychomycosis, hyperkeratosis is usually seen with longitudinal streaks, indicating the pattern of fungal invasion [25]. Contact dermatitis of the nail bed may also result in subungual hyperkeratosis; however, this most frequently involves the first three digits in the dominant hand [25]. In pityriasis rubra pilaris and/or lichen planus, other cutaneous or nail findings may suggest the diagnosis [25] (Fig. 11.11).

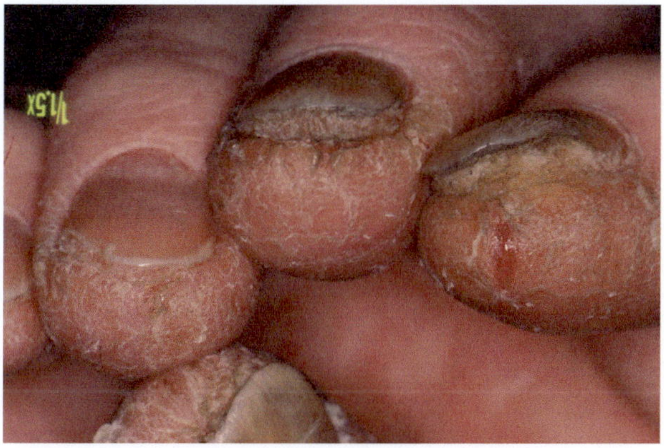

Fig. 11.10 Subungual hyperkeratosis in eczema

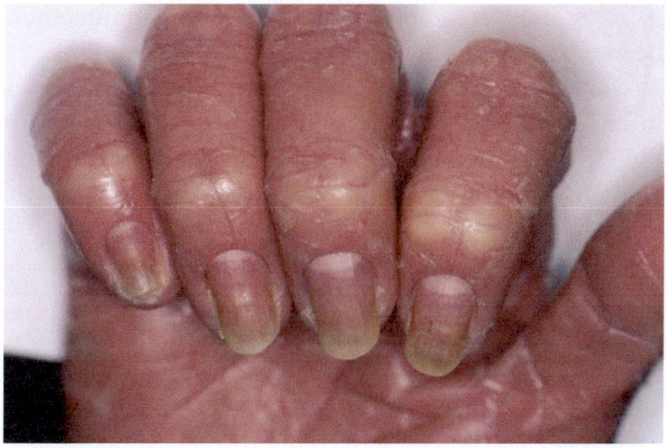

Fig. 11.11 Nail findings in pityriasis rubra pilaris

11.5 Splinter Hemorrhages

Several conditions, other than psoriasis, may cause distal splinter hemorrhages. The most common is trauma (Fig. 11.12); other acute traumatic sequelae may include subungual hematomas and nail shedding [26]. Distal splinter hemorrhages can also be found in onychomycosis and eczema [16].

Proximal splinters are very rare and may be indicative of systemic disorders, including infective endocarditis, renal or pulmonary disease, diabetes mellitus, vasculitis, and antiphospholipid syndrome [27–30]. Pain can help distinguish a systemic etiology, but may not be consistently present [31]. Cholesterol crystal embolization has also been reported in a patient with splinter hemorrhages of multiple finger and toenails [32]. Hemodialysis and peritoneal dialysis have also been identified as causes of splinter haemorrhages, with peritoneal dialysis reported as the most frequent factor in a cohort of patients with splinter hemorrhages [29, 33, 34].

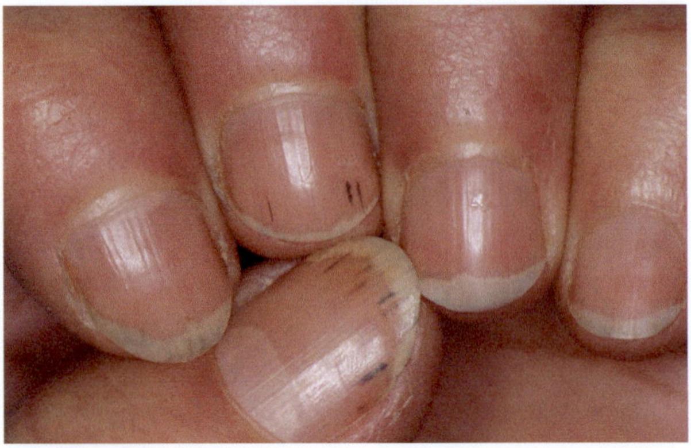

Fig. 11.12 Traumatic splinter hemorrhages

Drug-induced splinter hemorrhages in conjunction with onycholysis have also been reported after tetracycline use [35].

Splinter hemorrhages can also be found in healthy individuals, more frequently in males [27, 36]. When seen in females, they are often limited to a single digit [36–38]. Additionally, splinter hemorrhages are frequently seen in elderly patients who are more susceptible to nail damage.

11.6 Other Findings

Other nail findings, such as the "oil-drop sign" and red spots in the lunula, are more specific for psoriatic nail disease and can be used to help distinguish psoriasis from other dermatoses [39, 40]. This discoloration, along with pitting and nail plate crumbling, is virtually diagnostic of psoriasis [41].

Summary for the Clinician

The differential diagnosis of nail psoriasis includes nail abnormalities caused by traumatic, dermatological, and systemic disorders. Onychomycosis is more common in psoriatic nails and a diagnosis of onychomycosis does not exclude psoriasis.

References

1. Scher RK. Psoriasis of the nail. Dermatol Clin. 1985;3:387–94.
2. Lavaroni G, Kokelj F, Pauluzzi P, Trevisan G. The nails in psoriatic arthritis. Acta Derm Venereol Suppl (Stockh). 1994;186:113.
3. Tan ES, Chong WS, Tey HL. Nail psoriasis: a review. Am J Clin Dermatol. 2012;13:375–88. doi:10.2165/11597000-000000000-00000.
4. Jadhav VM, Mahajan PM, Mhaske CB. Nail pitting and onycholysis. Indian J Dermatol Venereol Leprol. 2009;75:631–3. doi:10.4103/0378-6323.57740.

5. Jiaravuthisan MM, Sasseville D, Vender RB, Murphy F, Muhn CY. Psoriasis of the nail: anatomy, pathology, clinical presentation, and a review of the literature on therapy. J Am Acad Dermatol. 2007;57:1–27. doi:10.1016/j.jaad.2005.07.073.
6. Baran R, Dawber RPR. The nail in dermatologic diseases. In: Baran R, RPR D, editors. Diseases of nail and their management. 2nd ed. Oxford: Blackwell Scientific Publications; 1994. p. 135–73.
7. Singh SK. Finger nail pitting in psoriasis and its relation with different variables. Indian J Dermatol. 2013;58:310–2. doi:10.4103/0019-5154.113955.
8. Tosti A, Piraccani B. Dermatologic diseases. In: Scher RK, editor. Nails diagnosis, therapy and surgery. 3rd ed. Philadelphia: Saunders; 2005. p. 116.
9. Baran R, Dawber RPR, Haneke E, Tosti A. Nail plate and soft tissue abnormalities. In: Baran R, Dawber RPR, Haneke E, Tosti A, Bristow I, Thomas L, et al., editors. A text atlas of nail disorders – techniques in investigation and diagnosis. London: Taylor & Francis; 2003.
10. Tosti A, Morelli R, Bardazzi F, Peluso AM. Prevalence of nail abnormalities in children with alopecia areata. Pediatr Dermatol. 1994;11:112–5.
11. Yung A, Johnson P, Goodfield MJ. Isotretinoin-induced elkonyxis. Br J Dermatol. 2005;153:671–2. doi:10.1111/j.1365-2133.2005.06782.x.
12. Greene RA, Scher RK. Nail changes associated with diabetes mellitus. J Am Acad Dermatol. 1987;16:1015–21.
13. Piraccani B, Iorizzo M. Diseases of the nails. In: Rakel R, Bope E, editors. Conn's current therapy 2008. Philadelphia: Saunders Elsevier; 2008.
14. Daniel 3rd CR, Iorizzo M, Piraccini BM, Tosti A. Simple onycholysis. Cutis. 2011;87:226–8.
15. Dawber RP, Samman PD, Bottoms E. Fingernail growth in idiopathic and psoriatic onycholysis. Br J Dermatol. 1971;85:558–60.
16. Tosti A, Piraccani BM. Nail disorders. In: Dermatology. Bolognia Jl, Jorizzo JL, Schaffer JV , (eds), Mosby Elsevier 2012. cap. 70:1019–36.
17. Natarajan V, Nath AK, Thappa DM, Singh R, Verma SK. Coexistence of onychomycosis in psoriatic nails: a descriptive study. Indian J Dermatol Venereol Leprol. 2010;76:723. doi:10.4103/0378-6323.72468.
18. Sigurgeirsson B, Steingrimsson O. Risk factors associated with onychomycosis. J Eur Acad Dermatol Venereol. 2004;18:48–51.
19. Kacar N, Ergin S, Ergin C, Erdogan BS, Kaleli I. The prevalence, aetiological agents and therapy of onychomycosis in patients with psoriasis: a prospective controlled trial. Clin Exp Dermatol. 2007;32:1–5. doi:10.1111/j.1365-2230.2006.02215.x.
20. Minisini AM, Tosti A, Sobrero AF, Mansutti M, Piraccini BM, Sacco C, et al. Taxane-induced nail changes: incidence, clinical presentation and outcome. Ann Oncol. 2003;14:333–7.
21. Baran R, Juhlin L. Drug-induced photo-onycholysis. Three subtypes identified in a study of 15 cases. J Am Acad Dermatol. 1987;17:1012–6.
22. Baran R, Juhlin L. Photoonycholysis. Photodermatol Photoimmunol Photomed. 2002;18:202–7.
23. Tosti A, Baran R, Dawber RPR. The nail in systemic diseases and drug induced changes. In: Baron R, Dawber RPR, editors. Diseases of the nail and their management. 2nd ed. Oxford: Blackwell Scientific Publications; 1994. p. 175–261.
24. Davies MG, McGavin CR. Onycholysis in sarcoidosis – a previously undescribed association. Br J Dermatol. 1996;135:340.
25. Tosti A, Daniel R, Piraccani B, Iorizzo M. Color atlas of nails. 1st ed. Berlin/Heidelberg/New York: Springer; 2009.
26. Mortimer PS, Dawber RP. Trauma to the nail unit including occupational sports injuries. Dermatol Clin. 1985;3:415–20.
27. Saladi RN, Persaud AN, Rudikoff D, Cohen SR. Idiopathic splinter hemorrhages. J Am Acad Dermatol. 2004;50:289–92. doi:10.1016/j.jaad.2003.07.012.
28. Frances C, Piette JC, Saada V, Papo T, Wechsler B, Chosidow O, et al. Multiple subungual splinter hemorrhages in the antiphospholipid syndrome: a report of five cases and review of the literature. Lupus. 1994;3:123–8.
29. Kilpatrick ZM, Greenberg PA, Sanford JP. Splinter hemorrhages – their clinical significance. Arch Intern Med. 1965;115:730–5.

30. Kimyai-Asadi A, Usman A, Milani F. Cutaneous manifestations of marantic endocarditis. Int J Dermatol. 2000;39:290–2.
31. Scher RK, Daniel R. Nails: therapy, diagnosis, surgery. Philadelphia: W.B. Sanders Company; 1990.
32. Turakhia AK, Khan MA. Splinter hemorrhages as a possible clinical manifestation of cholesterol crystal embolization. J Rheumatol. 1990;17:1083–6.
33. Blum M, Aviram A. Splinter hemorrhages in patients receiving regular hemodialysis. JAMA. 1978;239:47.
34. Kelly MP, Kight MA, Castillo S. Trophic implications of altered body composition observed in or near the nails of hemodialysis patients. Adv Ren Replace Ther. 1998;5:241–51.
35. Sanders CV, Saenz RE, Lopez M. Splinter hemorrhages and onycholysis: unusual reactions associated with tetracycline hydrochloride therapy. South Med J. 1976;69:1090–2.
36. Monk BE. The prevalence of splinter haemorrhages. Br J Dermatol. 1980;103:183–5.
37. Miller A, Vaziri ND. Recurrent atraumatic subungual splinter hemorrhages in healthy individuals. South Med J. 1979;72:1418–20.
38. Robertson JC, Braune ML. Splinter haemorrhages, pitting, and other findings in fingernails of healthy adults. Br Med J. 1974;4:279–81.
39. Kouskoukis CE, Scher RK, Ackerman AB. The "oil drop" sign of psoriatic nails. A clinical finding specific for psoriasis. Am J Dermatopathol. 1983;5:259–62.
40. van der Velden HM, Klaassen KM, van de Kerkhof PC, Pasch MC. Fingernail psoriasis reconsidered: a case-control study. J Am Acad Dermatol. 2013;69:245–52. doi:10.1016/j.jaad.2013.02.009.
41. Zaias N. Psoriasis of the nail. A clinical-pathologic study. Arch Dermatol. 1969;99:567–79.

Onychomycosis and Psoriasis

12

Bianca Maria Piraccini, Aurora Alessandrini,
and Carlton Ralph C. Daniel III

Contents

Key Features

- Onychomycosis and psoriasis are common diseases in the general population, and psoriasis may affect the nails.
- Several psoriatic nail features, like hyperkeratosis and onycholysis, may morphologically resemble onychomycosis.
- A differential diagnosis between the two diseases is difficult.
- Both disorders may coexist in the same nail.
- Mycological tests are often needed to do the correct diagnosis.

B.M. Piraccini, MD, PhD (✉) • A. Alessandrini, MD
Division of Dermatology, Department of Specialized, Experimental and Diagnostic Medicine, University of Bologna, Bologna, Italy
e-mail: biancamaria.piraccini@unibo.it; aurora.alessandrini@alice.it

C.R.C. Daniel III, MD
Clinical Professor of Dermatology, University of Mississippi Medical Center, University of Alabama, Birmingham, AL, USA
e-mail: crd322@aol.com

D. Rigopoulos, A. Tosti (eds.), *Nail Psoriasis: From A to Z*,
DOI 10.1007/978-3-319-08810-5_12

12.1 Introduction

Onychomycosis is the most frequent cause of abnormality of the nail unit, and it is responsible for about 50 % of all consultations for nail disorders. Onychomycosis has been reported as a gender- and age-related disease, being more prevalent in males and increasing with age in both genders [1]. In the elderly, onychomycosis may have an incidence >40 % [2]. Predisposing factors are diabetes mellitus, nail trauma, peripheral arterial disease, and immunosuppression due to HIV or immunosuppressive agents.

Psoriasis is a common skin disorder, occurring in about 2 % of the general population. The prevalence of nail involvement varies between 15 and 79 % of cases, with an estimated lifetime incidence of 80–90 % [3]; hands are more frequently affected than the feet, and usually more than one nail is involved.

Several psoriatic nail features, such as hyperkeratosis or onycholysis, may morphologically resemble onychomycosis, and a differential diagnosis between the two diseases often requires mycological tests. However, both disorders may be present in the same nail, especially toenails.

The prevalence of onychomycosis in psoriatic patient is still unclear and debated.

12.2 Onychomycosis

In most cases, onychomycosis is caused by anthropophilic dermatophytes of the genus *Trichophyton*; particularly, *Trichophyton rubrum* is the most common cause, followed by *Trichophyton interdigitale*. The non-dermatophyte molds can be primary pathogens, with prevalence figures ranging from 1.5 to 22 % in the world [4, 5]. *Scopulariopsis brevicaulis*, *Fusarium* spp., and *Aspergillus* spp. are the most common non-dermatophyte molds isolated in onychomycosis, usually located in the toenails [6]. Other molds that have been isolated include *Acremonium* spp., *Alternaria* spp., *Scytalidium* spp., and other less frequent species [7]. Yeasts represent a last common cause of nail fungal infection, and *Candida albicans* and *Candida parapsilosis* are the two most common species. They are seen in immunodepressed and diabetic patients.

There are different clinical types of onychomycosis, depending on the modality of nail invasion by the fungus.

12.2.1 Distal and Lateral Subungual Onychomycosis (DLSO)

DLSO is the most common type of onychomycosis and is characterized by a fungal invasion starting from the lateral or distal sites of the nail plate. The affected nails usually show subungual hyperkeratosis, onycholysis, and white or yellow discoloration (Figs. 12.1 and 12.2). Similar symptoms are commonly observed in toenail psoriasis (Figs. 12.3 and 12.4). Infrequently, brown, black, or orange discoloration may also be seen. In some cases, longitudinal streaks of the nail are present, called dermatophytoma: this entity may require excision or debulking of the area and systemic treatment.

DLSO usually affects one or both the great toenails and is also usually associated with tinea pedis (Fig. 12.5). The presence of tinea pedis is suggestive for onychomycosis and is easy to differentiate from psoriasis of the sole (Fig. 12.6).

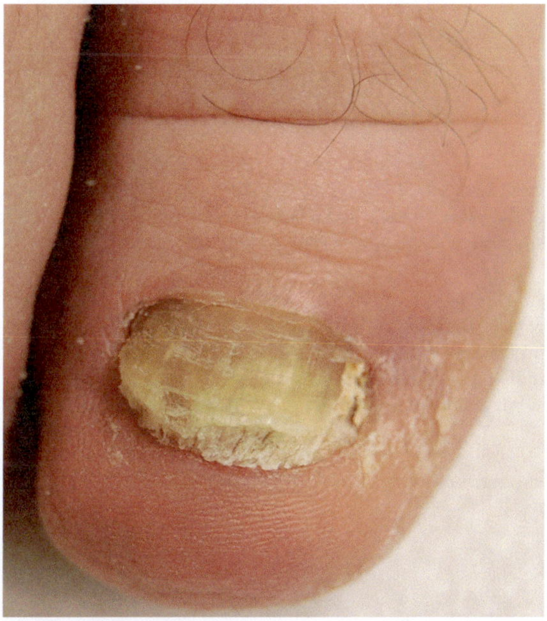

Fig. 12.1 Distal and lateral subungual onychomycosis (DLSO): onycholysis and subungual hyperkeratosis

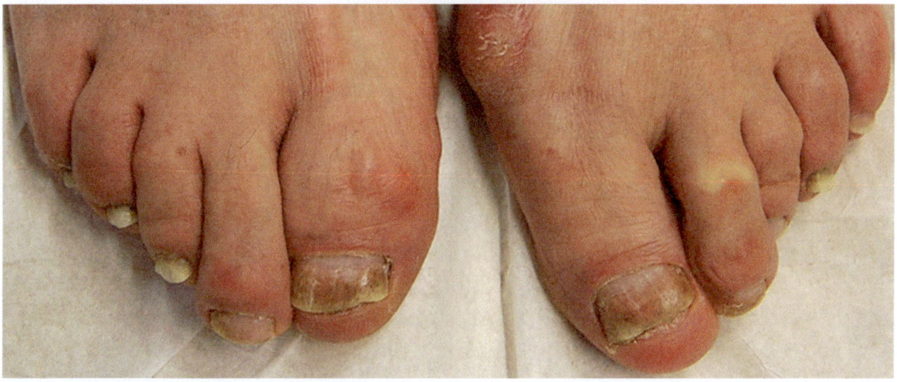

Fig. 12.2 Distal and lateral subungual onychomycosis (DLSO): onycholysis and subungual hyperkeratosis may involve several toenails

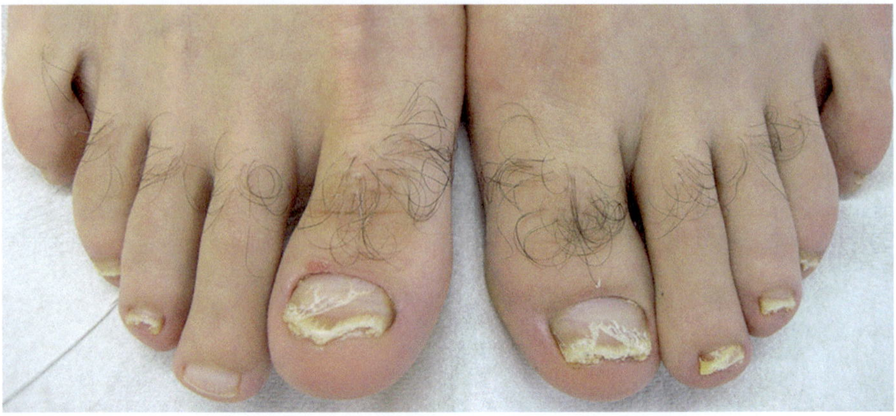

Fig. 12.3 Nail psoriasis: in the toenails, the most common symptoms are due to nail bed involvement with distal onycholysis and subungual hyperkeratosis. Note nail plate surface abnormalities of the great toenails and a small plaque of psoriasis in the proximal nail fold of the right toe, both suggestive for psoriasis but scarcely noticeable

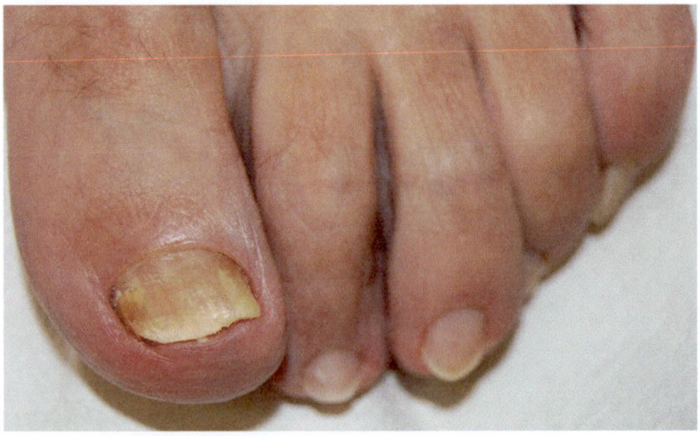

Fig. 12.4 Toenail psoriasis producing symptoms indistinguishable from distal subungual onychomycosis

12.2.2 Superficial Onychomycosis (SO)

SO can present with superficial patches or transverse striae and may arise from the superficial nail plate or emerge from the proximal nail fold. In the classic form (white superficial onychomycosis), dermatophytes colonize the most superficial layers of the nail plate without penetrating it. The affected nail presents multiple friable white opaque spots in a patchy distribution that can be easily scraped away. This form is due to dermatophytes, mainly *T. interdigitale*, and usually responds to topical treatment. In contrast, the striate form, when the infection emerges from the proximal nail fold and with deep penetration of the nail plate, is usually due to non-dermatophytes or may be caused by *T. rubrum* in young children, and oral therapy is usually necessary.

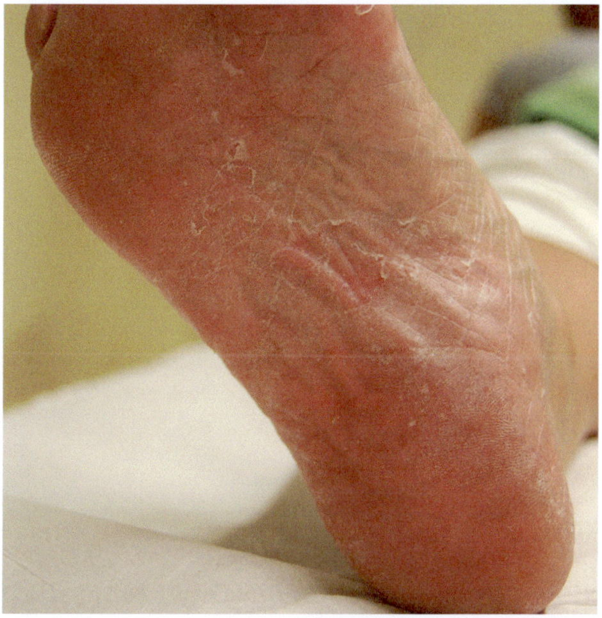

Fig. 12.5 Tinea pedis moccasin-type due to *Trichophyton rubrum*: diffuse scaling of the plantar skin without inflammatory signs

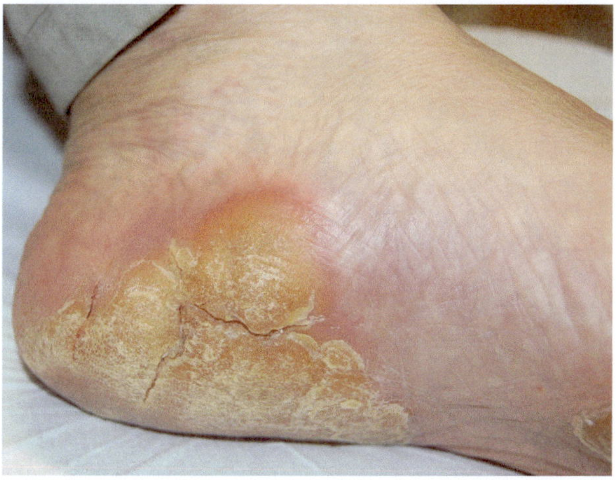

Fig. 12.6 Plantar psoriasis: the skin is intensely inflamed with severe thickening of the horny layer that leads to fissuring and pain

12.2.3 Endonyx Onychomycosis

Endonyx onychomycosis is characterized by massive nail plate parasitization in the absence of nail bed invasion. Clinically, the affected nail may show lamellar splitting and a milky white discoloration. The nail plate is firmly attached to the nail bed, and there is no nail bed hyperkeratosis or onycholysis. This type of infection is very rare and seen with *T. soudanense* or *T. violaceum*.

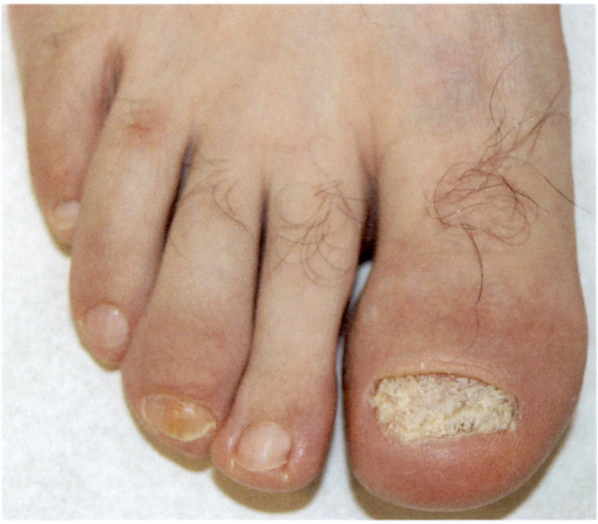

Fig. 12.7 Psoriasis of the nail matrix: the first toenail is crumbling due to severe nail fragility. Note the oil drop patch of the third toenail and the psoriatic arthropathy of the 1st digit

12.2.4 Proximal Subungual Onychomycosis (PSO)

PSO is characterized by a primitive invasion of the nail matrix keratogenous zone through the proximal nail fold horny layer. Fungal elements are typically located in the ventral nail plate; a proximal leukonychia that progresses distally with nail growth can be seen. Among the dermatophytes, these infections are usually caused by *T. rubrum* and are very rare. PSO is, on the other hand, a typical presentation of non-dermatophyte mold onychomycosis, where it is typically associated with periungual inflammation.

12.2.5 Mixed Pattern Onychomycosis

Many times different patterns of infection may be seen in the same patient. The most common of these are PSO with superimposed SO or DLSO with SO.

12.2.6 Total Dystrophic Onychomycosis (TDO)

TDO is the end stage of onychomycosis and can result from DLSO as well as PSO. The nail plate, in these cases, is fragile and crumbling and the underlying nail bed is thickened. This type of onychomycosis should be differentiated from psoriasis of the nail matrix, which produces diffuse nail plate fragility and crumbling (Fig. 12.7).

12.3 Diagnosis and Treatment of Onychomycosis

The clinical diagnosis of onychomycosis should be confirmed my mycology. A mycological exam is composed of two parts: the direct microscopic exam and culture. For the former, we have to display adequate material, previously collected from the affected nail and immersed in a solution of KOH 20–40 %, on a slide and then we observe under the microscope the characteristic aspects. With this examination, we do not know which pathogens cause the onychomycosis, so culture is the best option for a more specific diagnosis. Nail clippings can be utilized for diagnosing onychomycosis, with PAS stain that easily allows visualization of fungal hyphae. PCR techniques are a possible tool as well, but not yet developed to be utilized as routine diagnostic technique.

Confocal laser-scanning microscopy (CLSM) is an emerging technique particularly of interest in the diagnosis of nail disorders [8]. The aspect of dermatophytes can be easily observed in nail plate as a network of lengthy structures with high reflection and the typical shape of hyphae: the CLSM aspect of yeasts has been reported only by Arrese et al. [9], while molds have not been described yet in nails.

The difficulty in treating onychomycosis results from the deep-seated nature of the infection within the nail unit and the inability of the drugs to effectively reach all sites. Present treatment options include both oral and topical drugs, with oral therapies giving better outcomes.

The two most commonly used topical antifungal agents are amorolfine 5 % nail lacquer and ciclopirox 8 % nail lacquer. Amorolfine nail lacquer is applied once a week, whereas ciclopirox nail lacquer is applied daily. Nail lacquers are effective as monotherapy in the treatment of superficial onychomycosis and of distal subungual onychomycosis, limited to less than 50 % of the distal nail [10, 11]. Treatment duration should be at least 6–12 months. Nail lacquers are also utilized in combination with systemic antifungals [12] or nail avulsion in severe onychomycosis to reduce duration of treatment and increase cure rate [13].

Treatments with photodynamic therapy (PDT) using photosensitizers may also prove to be effective treatment options in the future [14]. Laser therapy is also currently being researched and may be effective in the treatment of onychomycosis. FDA-approved lasers for onychomycosis include carbon dioxide laser, ND: YAG laser, and the diode 870 nm, 930 nm laser.

Distal subungual onychomycosis that involves greater than 50 % of the nail, proximal subungual onychomycosis, and deeply infiltrating white superficial onychomycosis require systemic therapy [15]. Systemic treatment with terbinafine or itraconazole produces mycological cure in more than 90 % of fingernail infections and in about 80 % of toenail infections. These success rates can be increased by associating a topical treatment with a nail lacquer. Terbinafine can be administered as a continuous therapy at 250 mg per day for 12 weeks or an intermittent regimen of 2 pulses of 250 mg/day for 4 weeks on and 4 weeks off [16]. Itraconazole is administered as pulse therapy at the dosage of 200 mg twice a day for 1 week a month. The treatment duration is 2 months for fingernails and 3 months for toenails. Sequential treatment with itraconazole and terbinafine has been utilized to increase cure rates. Fluconazole is also used in dermatophyte onychomycosis but is less effective. Actually, in patients unable to tolerate other oral antifungal agents, the recommended dosage is 150–300 mg weekly for more than 6 months, especially for toenails [17].

12.4 Prevalence of Onychomycosis in Psoriatic Nails: Discussion

As mentioned, many psoriatic nail features may resemble onychomycosis, and a clinical differentiation between the two entities is difficult. In particular, in the toenails, both psoriasis and onychomycosis may produce onycholysis and subungual hyperkeratosis as the only manifestations, making differential diagnosis very difficult. Although diagnostic techniques, like direct microscopy and fungal culture, or nail clipping are often needed, there are some clinical clues that can help in the distinction between the two diseases. Onychomycosis tends to involve one or both great toenails, while nail psoriasis tends to affect at least several toenails. The fingernails may show typical signs of nail psoriasis and the disease may affect other skin sites, usually the scalp. Tinea pedis and psoriasis of the soles produce different signs. In the fingernails, differential diagnosis between nail psoriasis and onychomycosis may be difficult when one or a few nails are involved and the main sign is nail plate crumbling and whitening. This is in our experience a possible presentation of both diseases in the elderly.

Moreover, onychomycosis and psoriasis may coexist in the same nail, as both are frequent disorders in the general population (Table 12.1).

During the past decades, several studies were conducted to gain knowledge on the prevalence of onychomycosis in patients with nail psoriasis: the study protocols vary considerably in the literature and data are heterogeneous and ambiguous. The same lack of uniformity was found in reports about the involved pathogens.

Klaassen et al. [3] in a recent study performed a systemic review of all studies investigating this association, founding only ten articles considered appropriate for inclusion (Table 12.2). The topic is debated since the 1980s (two studies), while two studies were published in the 1990s and the remaining ones between 2000 and 2012. The majority of studies were performed in European countries.

Considering all studies individually, the prevalence of onychomycosis in nail psoriasis varied from 4.6 to 63.1 % compared to 2.4–66 % prevalence in the controls. Three studies concluded that a patient with nail psoriasis has a higher possibility to develop onychomycosis compared with healthy controls, and the remaining seven studies found no significant differences between patients and healthy controls.

In a study [18], the authors evaluated the prevalence of toenail onychomycosis in psoriatic patient and non-psoriatic patients attending dermatologists' offices, in which

Table 12.1 Psoriasis versus onychomycosis

Look for typical symptoms (pitting, salmon patches) in the fingernails
Look at the scalp or intergluteal clefts for psoriasis
History of spontaneous improvement and relapses suggests psoriasis
Presence of longitudinal streaks suggests onychomycosis
Potassium hydroxide (KOH) tests and culture are mandatory
Remember that both may present in the same nail, especially toenails

Table 12.2 Characteristics of the ten studies included in this chapter

Study	Country	Publication date	Pts, *n*	Ctr, *n*	Source	Selected patients	Location nail clipping
Gupta et al.	Canada/America	1997	561	922	Outpatients	Psoriasis	Toenail
Hamnerius et al.	Sweden	2004	239	245	Outpatients	Psoriasis	Toenail
Larsen et al.	Denmark	2003	79	142	Inpatients	Psoriasis	Both
Leibovici et al.	Israel	1998	113	102	In and out patients	Psoriasis	Toenail
Kacar et al.	Turkey	2006	168	164	Outpatients	Psoriasis	Both
Pawlaczyck et al.	Poland	2007	481	3,986	Outpatient	Psoriasis	Both
Staberg et al.	Denmark	1983	78	41	Outpatients	Psoriasis	Both
Stander et al.	Germany	2001	250	102	Outpatients	Psoriasis	Both
Szepes	Hungary	1986	137	341	Outpatients	Psoriasis	Both
Zawirska et al.	Poland	2006	70	30	Inpatients	Psoriasis	Toenails

onychomycosis was not a referring diagnosis. They found toenail onychomycosis in 13 % of psoriatic individuals; the frequency of fungal nail infection in patients suffering from psoriasis with the presence of nail abnormalities was even higher and reached 27 %; the pathogens were dermatophytes (*T. rubrum* and *T. mentagrophytes*). The authors concluded that the prevalence of onychomycosis of the toenails in psoriatic subjects was significantly higher than in non-psoriatic population.

Other studies did not confirm such a result: Hamnerius et al. [19] evaluated the frequency of tinea pedis and toenail onychomycosis in patients with psoriasis. They observed a low frequency of onychomycosis of the toenails in psoriatic patients: the difference between patients and healthy controls was not statistically significant, so they affirmed that there is no altered susceptibility to onychomycosis in psoriatic patients.

The pathogens more often responsible of onychomycosis in psoriatic patient with nail involvement were a discussed topic too [3]: yeast and/or non-dermatophyte molds were found more common in psoriatic than in normal nails in five studies and dermatophytes were most frequently found in three studies. In particular, dermatophytes seem to be the most common causative pathogens of onychomycosis of the toenails in psoriatic patients, while yeast are the most common pathogens of onychomycosis of the fingernails in these patients.

In the study of Stander et al. [20], in which 250 psoriatic patients with and without nail changes and 102 healthy controls were enrolled, yeast were more commonly present in involved psoriatic nails (23.9 %) than in psoriatics without nail changes (6.1 %) and in control group (6.9 %). Other authors [21, 22] stated that yeast more commonly affects nail plates with morphological abnormalities in the course of psoriasis.

A recent report by Martini et al. [23] described an interesting case of a nail psoriasis masqueraded by secondary infection of *Rhodotorula mucilaginosa*, a yeast that rarely causes onychomycosis in immunocompetent people. A 38-year-old man presented with nail dystrophy of all fingernails: the exams showed *R. mucilaginosa* as the causative agent, but after 2 months there was no clinical improvement with antimycotic therapy, so they performed a nail matrix biopsy of a toenail that showed an underlying nail psoriasis, successfully treated with oral acitretin e topical calcipotriol/betamethasone cream. In this case, probably nail dystrophy due to psoriasis constituted a predisposing factor for fungal superinfection.

Klaassen et al. [3] noted that in every study different methods of case/control identification were used and many different criteria like age and site of nail psoriasis were evaluated: this is the reason why the authors reported a very wide variation of onychomycosis prevalence in psoriatic patients.

Also the vulnerability of psoriatic nails for fungal invasion is discussed. Kacar et al. [24] in a study on the prevalence of onychomycosis in psoriatic patients stated that nail psoriasis constitutes a risk factor not for onychomycosis but only specifically for dermatophytic nail infections, because the disintegrated keratinocytes due to psoriasis may constitute a suitable environment for dermatophytes.

Larsen et al. [25] suggested that both the altered subungual tissue and the onycholysis may facilitate a yeast invasion. Some authors defend the hypothesis that morphological abnormalities of nail psoriasis act like predisposing factors for microorganisms' invasion. Another important aspect to evaluate is that psoriatic patients may be on immunosuppressive treatment (systemic or topical), and obviously this condition can facilitate the fungal infection of the nail [26, 27]. In addition, the abnormal capillary units in nail psoriasis impair the defense normally supplied by healthy hyponychium and weaken the defense system of the nail against invading microorganisms [28]. On the other hand, some authors noted that the immune response against microbial skin infections appears to be remarkably strong in psoriasis and that the fast turnover of the nail and the desquamation rate in these patients may constitute an effective defense against dermatophytes' invasion. Another study suggested that glycoprotein material, present in the nail, might be inhibitory to dermatophytes [29]. It seems logical though that psoriasis may break the seal between the nail plate and nail bed, thus allowing fungi into the nail unit.

Conclusion

There are still controversies whether psoriatic dystrophy of the nails is a predisposing factor for fungal infection. Most authors reported that the prevalence of onychomycosis in psoriatic patient is not higher than that in healthy population; however, yeast was more often isolated, probably as a contaminant agent. On the other hand, we should not forget that onychomycosis may occur in a patient with psoriasis.

In our experience, onychomycosis on psoriatic nails is uncommon and mycology is useful to distinguish between the two diseases more than to prove their association. The few cases of onychomycosis and psoriasis we have seen in our long-lasting experience were diagnosed or because the signs presented by the patient were diagnostic for both diseases or because when the onychomycosis was successfully cured by antifungal treatment, the nail maintained signs of psoriasis.

Because it is quite impossible to determine the presence of onychomycosis in psoriatic nails only by clinical examination, we suggest that all patients with

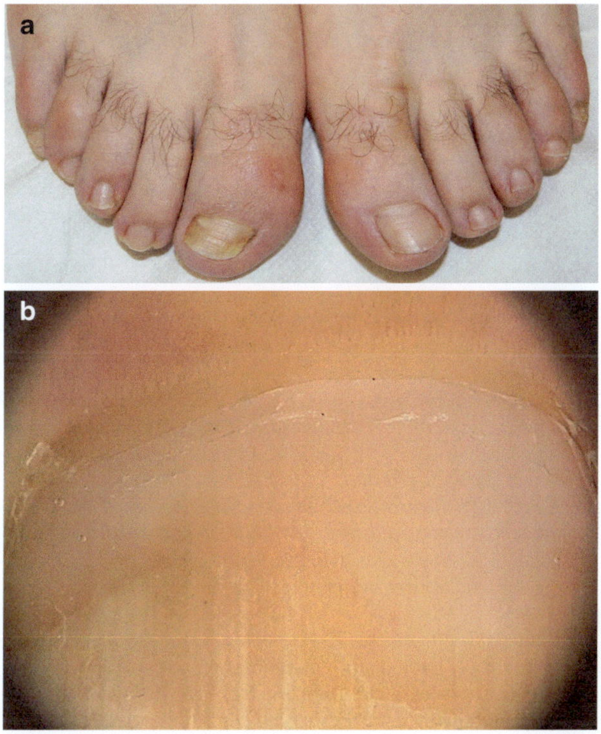

Fig. 12.8 (**a**) The first toe shows psoriasis of the nail and of the distal interphalangeal joint, which is visibly swollen. The nail shows mild onycholysis and orange discoloration. Onychoscopy (**b**) excludes onychomycosis showing proximal margin of the detachment

subungual hyperkeratosis or onycholysis should be tested with mycological examination for the presence of fungi in order to be treated with antifungal drugs. We have to remember that fungal infection may intensify nail psoriasis through the Koebner effect: prevent this adverse effect of the nail and adjacent skin is then possible.

Additionally, nail bed biopsies and dermoscopy may also be needed.

The use of dermoscopy in nail disorders is quite recent, known as "onychoscopy." The particular anatomy of the nail apparatus makes this technique not easy to perform and difficult to be interpreted, but onychoscopy can be very helpful to differentiate onychomycosis (in particular, DSO) from traumatic onycholysis. Even nail psoriasis has specific dermoscopic features. Although the final diagnosis relies on mycological results, there are three dermoscopic findings that are exclusive for onychomycosis: jagged edge of the proximal margin of the onycholytic area, with sharp structures (spikes) directed to the proximal fold, white-yellow longitudinal striae in the onycholytic nail plate, and an overall appearance of the affected nail plate in parallel bands of different colors, resembling aurora borealis [30]. In psoriatic patients, dermoscopy can be very useful when clinical features are not typical: we can see in fingernail onycholysis the erythematous border surrounding the distal edge of the detachment; the hyponychium can be observed too, showing irregularly distributed, dilated, tortuous, elongated capillaries [31]. However, in most of the cases, nail dermoscopy in toenail psoriasis only excludes onychomycosis showing onycholysis with a linear proximal border (Fig. 12.8a, b).

References

1. Heikkla H, Stubb S. The prevalence of onychomycosis in Finland. Br J Dermatol. 1995;133: 699–703.
2. Roseeuw D. Achilles foot screening project: preliminary results of patients screened by dermatologists. J Eur Acad Dermatol Venereol. 1999;12 Suppl 1:S6–9.
3. Klaassen KM, Dulak MG, van de Kerkhof PC, Pasch MC. The prevalence of onychomycosis in psoriatic patients: a systematic review. J Eur Acad Dermatol Venereol. 2014;28(5):533–41. doi:10.1111/jdv.12239.
4. Ramani R, Srinivas CR, Ramani A, Kumari TG, Shivananda PG. Molds in onychomycosis. Int J Dermatol. 1993;32:877–8.
5. Summerbell RC, Kane J, Krajden S. Onychomycosis, tinea pedis and tinea manuum caused by non-dermatophytic filamentous fungi. Mycoses. 1989;32:609–19.
6. Onsberg P. Scopulariopsis brevicaulis in nails. Dermatologica. 1980;161(4):259–64.
7. Degreef H. Onychomycosis. Br J Clin Pract Suppl. 1990;71:91–7.
8. Cinotti E, Fouilloux B, Perrot JL, Labeille B, Douchet C, Cambazard F. Confocal microscopy for healthy and pathological nail. J Eur Acad Dermatol Venereol. 2013. doi:10.1111/jdv.12330. [Epub ahead of print].
9. Arrese J-E, Quatresooz P, Piérard-Franchimont C, Piérard GE. Nail histomycology. Protean aspects of a human fungal bed. Ann Dermatol Venereol. 2003;130:1254–9.
10. Chang CH, Young-Xu Y, Kurth T, Orav JE, Chan AK. The safety of oral antifungal treatments for superficial dermatophytosis and onychomycosis: a meta-analysis. Am J Med. 2007;120: 791–8.
11. Baran R, Sigurgeirsson B, de Berker D, Kaufmann R, Lecha M, Faergemann J, Kerrouche N, Sidou F. A multicentre, randomized, controlled study of the efficacy, safety and cost-effectiveness of a combination therapy with amorolfine nail lacquer and oral terbinafine compared with oral terbinafine alone for the treatment of onychomycosis with matrix involvement. Br J Dermatol. 2007;157:149–57.
12. Tietz HJ, Hay R, Querner S, Delcker A, Kurka P, Merk HF. Efficacy of 4 weeks topical bifonazole treatment for onychomycosis after nail ablation with 40 % urea: a double-blind, randomized, placebo-controlled multicenter study. Mycoses. 2013;56:414–21.
13. Baran R, Tosti A, Hartmane I, Altmeyer P, Hercogova J, Koudelkova V, Ruzicka T, Combemale P, Mikazans I. An innovative water-soluble biopolymer improves efficacy of ciclopirox nail lacquer in the management of onychomycosis. J Eur Acad Dermatol Venereol. 2009;23: 773–81.
14. Piraccini BM, Rech G, Tosti A. Photodynamic therapy of onychomycosis caused by Trichophyton rubrum. J Am Acad Dermatol. 2008;59(5 Suppl):S75–6.
15. Lecha M, Effendy I, Feuilhade de Chauvin M, Di Chiacchio N, Baran R, Taskforce on Onychomycosis Education. Treatment options – development of consensus guidelines. J Eur Acad Dermatol Venereol. 2005;19 Suppl 1:25–33.
16. Gupta AK, Paquet M, Simpson F, Tavakkol A. Terbinafine in the treatment of dermatophyte toenail onychomycosis: a meta-analysis of efficacy for continuous and intermittent regimens. J Eur Acad Dermatol Venereol. 2013;27(3):267–72.
17. Gupta AK, Drummond-Main C, Paquet M. Evidence-based optimal fluconazole dosing regimen for onychomycosis treatment. J Dermatolog Treat. 2013;24:75–80.
18. Gupta AK, Lynde CW, Jain HC, et al. A higher prevalence of onychomycosis in psoriatics compared with non-psoriatics: multicentre study. Br J Dermatol. 1997;136:786–9.
19. Hamnerius N, Berglund J, Faergemann J. Pedal dermatophyte infection in psoriasis. Br J Dermatol. 2004;150:1125–8.
20. Ständer H, Ständer M, Nolting S. Häufigkeit des Pilzbefalles bei Nagelpsoriasis. Hautarzt. 2001;52:418–22.
21. Staberg B, Gammeltoft M, Onsberg P. Onychomycosis in patients with psoriasis. Acta Derm Venereol. 1983;63:436–8.

22. Szepes E. Mycotische Infektionen psoriatischer Nägel. Mykosen. 1986;29:82–4.
23. Martini K, Müller H, Huemer HP, Höpfl R. Nail psoriasis masqueraded by secondary infection with Rhodotorula mucilaginosa. Mycoses. 2013;56(6):690–2. doi:10.1111/myc.12091. Epub 2013 May 20.
24. Kacar N, Ergin S, Ergin C, Erdogan BS, Kaleli I. The prevalence, aetiological agents and therapy of onychomycosis in patients with psoriasis: a prospective controlled trial. Clin Exp Dermatol. 2007;32:1–5.
25. Larsen GK, Haedersdal M, Svejgaard EL. The prevalence of onychomycosis in patients with psoriasis and other skin diseases. Acta Derm Venereol. 2003;83:206–9.
26. Sanchez-Regana ML, Videla S, Villoria J, et al. Prevalence of fungal involvement in a series of patients with nail psoriasis. Clin Exp Dermatol. 2008;33:194–5.
27. Al-Mutairi N, Nour T, Al-Rqobah D. Onychomycosis in patients of nail psoriasis on biologic therapy: a randomized, prospective open label study comparing Etanercept, Infliximab and Adalimumab. Expert Opin Biol Ther. 2013;13(5):625–9. doi:10.1517/14712598.2013.783561. Epub 2013 Mar 26.
28. Leibovici V, Hershko K, Ingber A, Westerman M, Leviatan-Strauss N, Hochberg M. Increased prevalence of onychomycosis among psoriatic patients in Israel. Acta Derm Venereol. 2008; 88:31–3.
29. Zaias N. Psoriasis of the nail. A clinical-pathologic study. Arch Dermatol. 1969;99:567–79.
30. Piraccini BM, Balestri R, Starace M, Rech G. Nail digital dermoscopy (onychoscopy) in the diagnosis of onychomycosis. J Eur Acad Dermatol Venereol. 2013;27(4):509–13.
31. Piraccini BM, Bruni F, Starace M. Dermoscopy of non-skin cancer nail disorders. Dermatol Ther. 2012;25(6):594–602.

Treatment of Nail Psoriasis

13

Dimitrios Rigopoulos

Contents

Key Features

- Nail psoriasis treatment should be indivisualized.
- Management of the disease depends on the part of the nail which is affected.
- Despite the lack of evidence-based efficacy of topical treatment, it should be a choice for the clinician.
- When many nails are affected, systemic treatment should be used.

D. Rigopoulos, MD
Department of Dermatology, Athens University School of Medicine, Athens, Greece
e-mail: drigop@hol.gr

D. Rigopoulos, A. Tosti (eds.), *Nail Psoriasis: From A to Z*,
DOI 10.1007/978-3-319-08810-5_13

More treatment protocols have been introduced for psoriasis than virtually for all the rest of dermatology put together. Despite these recent therapeutic advances, management of nail psoriasis, a disease which is frequently overlooked, remains difficult, sometimes impractical, tiresome, and in some cases with an outcome which is unsatisfactory. The lack of guidelines and the low level of evidence that are available are more than obvious, so treating nail psoriasis is a difficult challenge that each clinician has to take up.

Management of nail psoriasis should be individualized (we always treat the patient and not the disease), and this depends on the part of the nail which is affected (location), association of skin and/or joint lesions, quality of life (if the disease is located on the fingernails), chariness of body systems, age and gender of the patient, and productivity or ability to work.

Before the introduction of any treatment, there are some general measures for the patients, for hand and nail care. These include the use of gloves better with cotton ones underneath (*for wet work and contact with irritant fluids*), use of nail moisturizers, avoidance of trauma (*over-rigorous manipulations*), and avoidance of tight or high heel shoes in order to avoid trauma of toenail which can act as a Koebner phenomenon and either increase existing nail psoriasis or lead to the appearance of the disease; patients should keep their nails short in order to prevent exacerbation of onycholysis, they should never extract debris from beneath the nail with an instrument, they should avoid nail biting, they are encouraged to use colored nail lacquer, they should avoid the use of nail polish removers with formaldehyde-acetone and toluene and also artificial nails, they should change occupation whenever of course this is possible and in mild disease they must be reassured from their consultant for the future, as their disease can improve spontaneously [1–6].

Topical treatment is indicated in mild nail psoriasis nonassociated with psoriatic arthritis, if only few nails are affected, if the nail bed is affected, when systemic treatment is not recommended, and in combination with systemic treatment. The clinician should keep in mind that topical treatment is not as efficient as on psoriatic skin, as the nail plate prevents drug penetration and that it takes a longer time for noticeable nail improvement (3–9 months), due to the slow growth rate of the nail. So topical treatment due to the abovementioned reasons can result in poor patient compliance.

If the clinical signs of the disease are due to the involvement of the nail matrix, then topical medication should be applied on the proximal nail fold, while if the signs indicate effect of psoriasis on the nail bed, then the onycholytic part of the nail should be removed before treatment; otherwise penetration of drugs used is limited or even absent.

Despite the lack of evidence-based efficacy of topical treatment and the fact that results are in some cases of poor quality, this does not mean that these treatments are not efficacious.

Topical treatment includes:

- Topical steroids
- Vitamin D analogues
- Tazarotene
- Fluorouracil
- Anthralin
- Tacrolimus

- Local PUVA
- Laser
- Photodynamic
- Combination treatment
- Miscellaneous

Concerning the topical use of 70 % oral cyclosporine solution with maize oil which was reported in the literature to be a safe, effective, and highly cosmetically accepted alternative treatment for nail psoriasis, this was never confirmed by other authors and in our experience it proved to be inefficacious, so it is already an abandoned modality [7].

13.1 Steroids

Topical steroids can be used in the form of creams or ointments, once or twice a day, with or without occlusion. Potent or superpotent steroids are usually used for a period of 4–6 months at the nail bed if onycholytic nail is clipped back or at the nail folds. Skin atrophy, telangiectasias on the surrounding skin, tachyphylaxis, and atrophy of the underlying phalanx (disappearing digit) can appear as side effects if their use is prolonged. Topical treatment with corticosteroids is unable to act properly in case of subungual hyperkeratosis. Therefore, nail debridement using 40 % urea under occlusion allows treatment of the nail bed after removal of the pathological area.

Considering the low cost and the advantages of new "modern" steroids with lower rate of adverse effects and the possibility for once-a-day application, topical steroids remain an excellent, possibly first-line treatment for psoriatic nail.

Intralesional use of steroids can also be used, and by certain physicians, this seems to be the treatment of choice despite the negative attitude of the patients in some cases, since it is a rather painful procedure. Triamcinolone acetonide solution is the most popular steroid, and it is used at different solution concentrations ranging from 2.5 to 5 mg/ml and quantity per site injected between 0.05 and 01 ml at up to four injection areas. Usually injections are performed with a 30 g needle locked to the syringe, monthly or bimonthly for 5–6 months at the proximal nail fold, as it is useful mainly in nail matrix psoriasis (pitting, nail plate crumbling). In cases of nail signs due to the affection of the nail bed, injections must be performed at the lateral nail folds in the nail bed [8, 9].

In one study a more potent triamcinolone acetonide solution (10 mg/ml) in a dosage of 0.1 ml was used for bimonthly injections with excellent results regarding subungual hyperkeratosis (100 % reduction), pitting (57.7 %), and onycholysis (40.5 %) [10]. The same concentration but with four 0.1 ml injections at the same time, which was repeated if needed after 2 months, was reported in another study which included 19 patients, with excellent results for subungual hyperkeratosis (100 %), ridging (94 %), and nail plate thickening (83 %) but not with onycholysis (50 %) and pitting (45 %) after 9.4 months of patient follow-up. Dermo-jet is a modality abandoned due to the sterilization problems of the apparatus and also the possibility of "splash back" of small quantities of blood at the time of injections [8]. There is also a case report of a patient forced to digit amputation after the use of Port-O-Jet (needleless high pressure injector) due to the development of epidermoid inclusion cysts after treatment [11]. Lidocaine 2.5 % and prilocaine 2.5 % in the form of a cream under occlusion or in the form of patches can be used 30–60 min prior the infusions in order to comfort patients before the injections and increase their compliance, or in some cases distal block anesthesia can be also used. Ice or refrigerant spray has also been reported in order to cool the digit and comfort the patient [12].

New forms of older drugs, such as steroids, *or new delivery systems* have been reported in the recent literature to be effective in treating nail psoriasis.

So, in three studies, one back in 1999 and two more recently published (2012), 8 % clobetasol nail lacquer used twice a week for 16 weeks has been reported to be effective and safe for both nail matrix and nail bed signs of psoriasis, and it can be considered a good option for topical therapy in the treatment of the disease [13–15]. The high steroid concentration and the lacquer vehicle ensure penetration of the drug through the nail plate and increased efficacy. Iontophoresis, a technique which uses a slight electric charge to enhance delivery of drugs through the skin, was used in order to increase dexamethasone absorption in patients with nail psoriasis. The method was used once every week and for 12 weeks. Twenty-seven patients were included in this open small study and NAPSI was the measuring system used for efficacy. According to the authors of the paper, 81 % improvement was reported in all patients who tolerated well the method [16].

13.2 Vitamin D Analogues (Calcipotriol-Tacalcitol)

Calcipotriol (synthetic Vitamin D analogue, which inhibits proliferation and differentiation of keratinocytes and also suppresses T-cell activity and cytokine production) has been used twice a day for 4–6 months, at the nail plate, the hyponychium, and the nail bed if onycholytic nail is clipped back and at the nail folds, with improvement mainly reported for hyperkeratosis. Tosti et al. reported a 49 % reduction of subungual hyperkeratosis after 5 months of application of calcipotriol, in a randomized double-blind study [17].

In another recently published study, 24 patients were also treated with calcipotriol twice a day without any occlusion, for 12 weeks. The medication was applied on the nail folds and the nail plate. Fingernails responded better than toenails, and hyperkeratosis, onycholysis, and discoloration were the symptoms that responded better [18]. Calcipotriol, 5 days week (weekdays) and clobetasol propionate 2 times a week (weekends), on the nail plate, nail folds and hyponychium, has been used with excellent results after 6 and 12 months of patient's evaluation (72 % improvement on the 6th month and 81 % after 12 months on the fingernails and 70 % which increased to 73 % at the toenails, on the same period of time) [19].

Calcipotriol was used twice a day (it was applied on the nail and the periungual tissues) in a study on 15 patients with pustular psoriasis, and it proved to be effective in 60 % (9/15) of them after 3–6 months of treatment [20]. In the same study, calcipotriol was used in 6 patients with pustular psoriasis who responded to systemic retinoid treatment (etretinate 0.5 mg/kg/daily or acitretin 0.5 mg/kg/day and with a mean duration of treatment of 6 months), as a maintenance treatment, and it proved to have prevented severe recurrences.

In all these studies, fingernails seem to respond better than toenails.

Tacalcitol (synthetic analogue of Vitamin D3 with hydroxylation in the position 24 instead of the position 25 as in Calcitriol) has been used successfully in the treatment of 15 patients with psoriatic onychodystrophy. Patients used the ointment once a day for 6 months and a significant improvement in all nail parameters (both nail matrix and nail bed signs) was reported by the authors [21].

13.3 Tazarotene

Tazarotene 0.1 % gel (synthetic retinoid which downregulates hyperproliferation of keratinocytes, differentiation, and inflammation) was applied on two target fingernails at bedtime one with and the other without occlusion in a randomized, vehicle-controlled, parallel-group trial including 31 patients. Patients were randomized to receive either the active gel or the vehicle, and they used this treatment for 21 weeks. Tazarotene resulted in significantly greater reduction of onycholysis (in the occluded and non-occluded nails) and pitting (in the occluded nails) [22]. Tazarotene 0.1 % gel was applied at bedtime without occlusion to the nail plate, the nail folds, and the periungual skin for 48 weeks, with 76 % of the patients showing a good to very good response. Fingernails responded better than toenails and tolerability was excellent (*mild erythema, peeling of the proximal nail fold, burning*) [23]. Tazarotene 0.1 % gel was also used in 23 patients while 23 more used clobetasol cream 0.05 % under occlusion for 12 weeks and were followed up for 12 more weeks. Statistical significant improvement of NAPSI score was reported for both groups, but at the end of the follow-up period, patients in the tazarotene group appeared with minor relapse rate concerning hyperkeratosis [24]. Tazarotene gel can cause mild skin irritation with burning sensation and desquamation of the area. In a small recently published study, six patients used, under occlusion every night and for 6 months, tazarotene 0.1 % hydrophilic ointment with a percentage improvement reaching 87.9 % at the end of treatment period [25].

13.4 Fluorouracil

Different results have been reported with the use of fluorouracil (it inhibits the thymidylate synthesis) either used alone as monotherapy (1 % or 5 % in different vehicles) or combined with urea 20 % or used in combination with urea and propylene glycol in the form of a solution. Subungual hyperkeratosis, onycholysis, and oil-spots are the symptoms with the greater efficacy after usually 4 months of treatment (one study showed increase of onycholysis). A high rate of nail loss, as well as hyperpigmentation and skin irritation, has been reported in all studies using fluorouracil [26–28].

13.5 Anthralin

Anthralin (possesses anti-inflammatory and antiproliferative properties) in a concentration ranging between 0.4 and 2 % in petrolatum applied once a day for 30 min and then rinsed off with plain water and for up to 5 months was used in a Japanese study and improvement was reported in almost 60 % of the patients regarding hyperkeratosis, onycholysis, and pitting. Reversible pigmentation of the nail plate was the main undesired effect [29].

13.6 Tacrolimus

Tacrolimus 0.1 % ointment (with immunosuppressive properties) was shown to be an effective and safe therapeutic option for the treatment of nail psoriasis used on 21 patients who applied the medication on the nail folds at bedtime, without occlusion for 12 weeks, in a left-right randomly used application of the drug. It has proven to be effective for both nail matrix and bed signs, only on the nails of the hand that used the medication. No topical or systemic side effects were reported by the patients [30].

Tacrolimus is a high molecular weight substance so one could raise the question of how does it penetrate the nail plate and the skin of the nail folds. The probable answer is that this happens due to its lipophilicity and the ointment formulation (it suspends the transungual and transcutaneous water transport so it increases the transungual drug penetration). These data should be confirmed by a double-blind study with a larger sample of patients.

13.7 Local Puva

In the literature there are only two papers, one published in 1977 and the other in 1987, reporting good response with local PUVA treatment of the psoriatic nails. A 1 % solution of 8-methoxypsoralen was applied at the proximal nail fold and then UVA was used two to three times per week. Onycholysis seemed to respond better than pitting [31, 32].

In a recent study using cadaveric nails, it was demonstrated that UVB is completely blocked by the nail plate while only a minimal amount of UVA penetrates it, so this might explain the minimal effect of PUVA on nail psoriasis and the lack of further interest of the clinicians [33].

13.8 Laser Treatment

Pulse Dye Laser (PDL) was found to be an effective and well-tolerated option in the treatment of both nail bed and nail matrix psoriasis on 20 patients, after 6 months of first treatment. No significant difference in terms of efficacy was found between the longer and shorter pulse duration treatment groups, and only a higher level of pain, statistically significant, was observed with the longer pulse duration [34]. On another study five patients were treated with PDL 595 nm, once a month for 3 months, and a statistical significant difference of NAPSI score was observed before and after treatment with better response for nail bed lesions (onycholysis and hyperkeratosis) [35]. In a recent case report, PDL 595 nm once monthly, for 3 months, proved also to be effective and safe for both nail matrix and nail bed signs of nail psoriasis [36].

13.9 Photodynamic Treatment

Photodynamic treatment (PDT) with the application on the nail plate of methylaminolaevulinic acid (MAL) under occlusion for 3 h, followed by PDL 595 nm irradiation (7 mm, 6 ms, 9 J/cm^2, three pulses on each nail) once a month for 6 months was compared with PDL 595 nm as monotherapy on the other hand of the same patient, with the same parameters. Fourteen patients were treated and the results show that both treatments are equally effective; thus, MAL does not increase the beneficial effect of PDL. Pain was not an important issue for the patients [37].

13.10 Combination Treatment

A combination of calcipotriol and betamethasone ointment, used at bedtime for 7 days a week and for a period of 12 weeks at the nail folds, the nail plate and the hyponychium with a mean 72 % NAPSI improvement mainly on hyperkeratosis and onycholysis, has also been reported in the literature [38] (Fig. 13.1a, b). Clobetasol 8 % nail lacquer has been used in combination with tacalcitol (synthetic vitamin D3

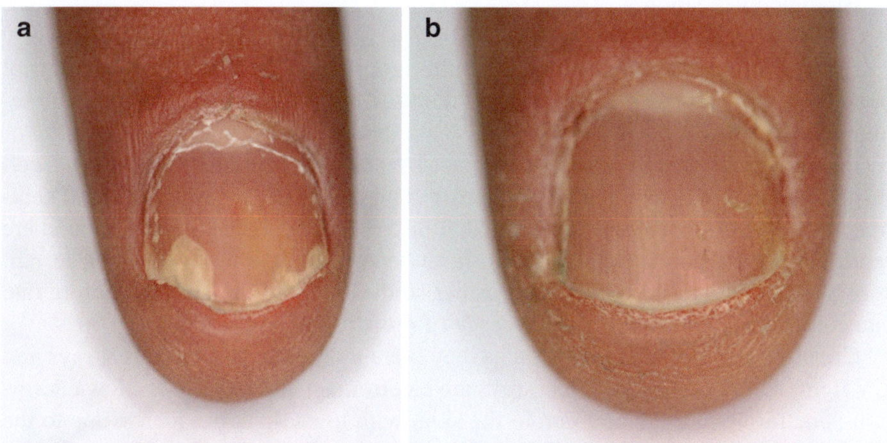

Fig. 13.1 (**a**) Before treatment. (**b**) Twelve weeks after treatment with calcipotriol and betamethasone ointment

analogue) ointment on 15 patients with both matrix and bed nail psoriasis. The lacquer was used at bedtime on weekends and tacalcitol on weekdays under occlusion, and this was for 6 months. NAPSI fell by 78 % compared to baseline while tolerability was excellent [39]. The efficacy of PDL plus topical tazarotene 0.1 % gel once a month for 6 months vs tazarotene 0.1 % gel alone in nail psoriasis was studied in a single-blind, intrapatient left-to-right study including 19 patients. The results of the study favor the combination in a significantly superior manner [40].

13.11 Miscellaneous

Based on the properties and its effectiveness in the management of nail splitting and nail brittleness when regularly applied on damaged nails, a non-drug, water-soluble nail lacquer, containing hydroxypropyl chitosan, which forms a film on the nail surface after application and evaporation of the solvent, was used in a studying order to improve nail psoriasis symptoms. Overall, 28 patients were included in the efficacy analysis, and at the end of the treatment period, results showed a 72 % reduction in pitting, 66 % reduction in leukonychia, 63 % reduction in onycholysis, and a reduction of 65 % in NAPSI score, compared to baseline [41].

Systemic treatment is indicated in nail psoriasis involving many or all nails, when it is associated with moderate or severe skin symptoms linked with or without arthritis and in cases of pustular psoriasis of the nail (acrodermatitis continua of Hallopeau).

Systemic treatment refers to the use of:

- Acitretin
- Cyclosporin A
- Methotrexate
- Biologic medication

Either as monotherapy or together with vigorous topical treatment (calcipotriol or steroids), in order to reduce dose and duration of systemic treatment or to maintain disease remission.

Fumaric acid esters (they probably act by skipping the Th1-dominated T-cell response in psoriasis to a Th2-like pattern and inhibition of the proliferation of keratinocytes), which are licensed in Germany for the treatment of skin psoriasis and are reported to have good response rates, have been also cited to be effective in nail psoriasis in just a case report [42]. Further studies are probably needed before one can come to a conclusion for the efficacy of this drug in nail psoriasis.

Grenz (means *border* in German as they were thought to be between X-rays and UV light in their biological effect) rays are electromagnetic radiation of low energy, non-penetrating more than 2 mm in the skin, with low efficacy evidence due to the small number of patients treated for nail psoriasis with this method. There are also concerns for the safety, as there probably is a risk for skin malignancy in the surrounding skin if, of course, these are used for a long period of time [43]. Superficial radiotherapy was also used in a limited number of patients with nail psoriasis, but with a temporary-only benefit [44]. Electron beams were used to treat 12 patients with nail psoriasis (0.75 Gy/week for 8 weeks) with temporary-only improvement (full relapse after 6 months in 6 patients and after one year in 9 patients) [45].

These treatment modalities are not used any more for psoriatic nail disease.

13.11.1 Acitretin

Acitretin is used in a dosage ranging between 0.2 and 0.3 mg/kg/day and, in cases lower than that, used in skin psoriasis in order to avoid side effects like nail fragility, reduction of nail thickness, pseudopyogenic-type granuloma, and anonychia-like lesions. Six months of treatment of 36 patients with low dose of acitretin (0.2–0.3 mg/kg/day) leads to 41 % reduction of NAPSI score (and 50 % in the mean NAPSI score of the target nail) in a study published by Tosti et al. [46]. Acitretin has also been used in association with urea nail lacquer in a 73-year-old female patient with an impressive finger- and toenail psoriasis, and after 6 months of treatment, excellent results have been reported [47].

Piraccini et al. have used acitretin 0.5 mg/kg/day to treat a small number of patients with pustular psoriasis of the nails with good response but with a high relapse rate [20].

13.11.2 Cyclosporin A

The efficacy of cyclosporin A (CyA) (it acts by inhibition of T-cell activity and decrease of inflammatory mediators) has been studied indirectly in studies using the medication for the treatment of skin psoriasis. In a multicenter study where 90 psoriasis patients with nail disease symptoms were included and the efficacy of CyA at a starting dosage of 3 mg/kg followed by either the increase of the dosage to 5 mg/kg/day where needed for 10 weeks and discontinuation thereafter or after the first 10 weeks the tapering of the dosage during the next 12 weeks, were studied for its efficacy on nail psoriasis. According to the authors of the study, in the first group there was a decrease of the nail involvement by 26.2 % and in the second group by 46.0 % [48]. In a recently published retrospective study, seven patients were treated for nail psoriasis with 3 mg/kg/day, and after 12 weeks, 37.9 % (23.0–52.9) reduction of NAPSI was observed; after 24 weeks of treatment the NAPSI score was reduced by 71.8 % [7–77] and at week 48 by 89.1 % (85.3–92.9) [49]. The same authors have reported long-term improvement of nail psoriasis symptoms, of both matrix and bed affection, in a series of 70 patients treated with 3 mg/kg of CyA for 8 weeks [50]. Another study included 54 patients with skin and nail psoriasis, and the patients were divided into two groups, one receiving CyA as monotherapy at a dosage ranging between 3.5 and 4.5 mg/kg/day and the other combining CyA 3.5–4.5 mg/kg/day with calcipotriol cream applied twice daily. After 12 weeks of treatment, the combination group of patients showed 79 % improvement of subungual hyperkeratosis, onycholysis, and pitting, while the monotherapy group showed 47.6 % reduction of the same symptoms. Twenty-four weeks after discontinuation of treatment 37 % of the patients in the combination group showed relapse while the percentage was 52.9 % in the monotherapy group [51]. In a study that included 16 patients with nail changes due to psoriasis, CyA in an initial dosage of 3 mg/kg/day and after improvement reduction to 1.5 mg/kg/day was administrated, with over 90 % of the patient being improved and satisfied, while in the period of follow-up (4–15 months), all the followed-up patients (7 patients) had no relapse [52]. In a one-blind randomized study, 17 patients with nail psoriasis received CyA 5 m/kg/day for 24 weeks, with a moderate result, in comparison with the other studies using the same high dosage and the same long period of time. There was a reduction of NAPSI up to 45.2 % for fingernails and 37.2 % for toenails and mainly referring to the nail bed signs [53].

From the majority of the abovementioned studies, it is clear that CyA is an effective treatment modality for nail psoriasis and since side effects reported in all studies are not serious, one could consider it also as a safe treatment.

13.11.3 Methotrexate

Only a small number of studies using methotrexate (MTX) to treat nail psoriasis exist. Low dose of MTX (5 mg/week) was reported to be efficient after 9 months for fingernails and 13 months for toenails, in a female 11-year-old patient with severe nail psoriasis affecting all 20 nails [54]. Reich et al. used MTX for nail psoriasis and reported a reduction of NAPSI 36.8 % after 24 weeks, increasing to 39.3 % after 52 weeks [55]. In a retrospective study [49], 9 patients were treated for nail psoriasis with MTX 5 mg/week as initial dosage and thereafter with 7.5–25 mg/week for 48 weeks, and a 7.3 % [3, 8–10] reduction of NAPSI was observed, after 12 weeks of treatment, which was increased to 30.8 % [2–43] at week 24 and to 34.9 % (21.9–48.0) at week 48. In a one-blind randomized study, 17 patients with nail psoriasis received MTX 15 mg/day for 24 weeks with a reduction of NAPSI up to 49.3 % for fingernails and 43.1 % for toenails and mainly referring to the nail matrix signs [53].

Intralesional MTX was used in one patient, with injections of 2.5 mg/week for 6 weeks and a significant reduction of subungual hyperkeratosis and pitting and the most important maintenance of the result for 2 years [56].

13.11.4 Biologics

Newer treatments for skin psoriasis include anti-TNFa (alefacept, fully human recombinant fusion protein; adalimumab, human monoclonal antibody; etanercept, fusion protein; infliximab, chimeric monoclonal antibody) and anti-IL-12,-23 drugs (briakinumab, human monoclonal antibody; ustekinumab, recombinant, completely human, monoclonal antibody). Most of these drugs have been studied for their efficacy on nail psoriasis, despite the lack of on-label indication.

A retrospective study was conducted based on the medical records of 12 patients treated with infliximab, 14 with adalimumab, and 13 with etanercept in daily practice [57]. The NAPSI was recorded at baseline, week 12, 24, and 48. At week 12, NAPSI was improved compared to baseline by 48.0 % (range: 40.2–66.6 %) with infliximab, 35.0 % (range: 25.0–52.6 %) with adalimumab, and 41.7 % (range: 39.5–46.4 %) with etanercept. At week 24, NAPSI was improved by 80.4 % (range: 66.6–90.2 %) with infliximab, 70.2 % (66.6–80.2 %) with adalimumab, and 76.1 % (62.5–85.5 %) with etanercept. At week 48, NAPSI was improved by 95.1 % (range: 89.5–97.3 %) with infliximab, 89.5 % (75.0–94.8 %) with adalimumab, and 92.8 % (84.3–96.0 %) with etanercept. NAPSI percentage improvement was statistically significant across follow-up period ($p=0.000$) for each anti-TNFa treatment, as well as among treatments at all time points (week 12, $p=0.000$; week 24, $p=0.001$; week 48, $p=0.000$). So, according to the authors of this study, all anti-TNFa agents result in a significant improvement of NAPSI score, with infliximab given the precedence and followed by etanercept and adalimumab.

Another recently published open-label retrospective study by Bardazzi et al. [58] considered patients affected by nail psoriasis and moderate to severe cutaneous disease. Medical records of 54 patients receiving biologics were analyzed. Eighteen of these were receiving etanercept, 16 adalimumab, 14 infliximab, and 6 ustekinumab. At week 36, 88.89 % of the etanercept patients, 93.75 % of the adalimumab, 85.71 % of the infliximab, and 83.33 % of the ustekinumab patients achieved NAPSI75, while improvement was seen starting on week 12 with all drugs.

The data from these two studies, confirm that all biologic agents are effective in treating nail psoriasis, almost at the same percentage.

Analysis of the efficacy of each biologic agent separately follows.

13.11.4.1 Alefacept

This drug was used intramuscularly and in a dosage of 15 mg/week, in a small study published in 2005 in 6 patients with nail disease. Despite the significant improvement reported by the authors (decrease of NAPSI score more than 30 %), we have to mention that this was seen in only three of these patients and that patients selected had mild psoriasis (NAPSI score below 7 in 67 % of them) [59].

In another small series of patients but with at least moderate nail disease (NAPSI score greater than 15), 2 patients were reported to improve, 2 remained unchanged, and in 1 patient the disease was aggravated, after 3 months treatment with alefacept, 15 mg weekly intramuscularly [60].

Fifteen patients were treated with alefacept, 15 mg weekly for 12 weeks, and in 39 % of them there was a reduction of NAPSI score after 12 weeks from the treatment discontinuation [61].

These are small clinical studies and one cannot come to a certain conclusion concerning the efficacy of this drug in nail psoriasis. Unfortunately the drug was discontinued after the cases of progressive multifocal leukoencephalopathy that were reported [62].

13.11.4.2 Etanercept

Five hundred sixty-four psoriasis patients were treated subcutaneously with either 25 mg etanercept twice/week for 54 weeks or 50 mg twice/week for 12 weeks and presented with NAPSI score improvement by 29 % at week 12, by 51 % at week 24, and complete resolution in 30 % of them at week 54 (169 patients) [63]. Sixty-nine patients with moderate to severe cutaneous and nail psoriasis received etanercept treatment with either 50 mg twice/week for 12 weeks followed by 50 mg once/week for 12 more weeks or 50 mg once/week for 24 weeks in an open randomized study. The primary endpoint was the improvement of NAPSI score on the target fingernail. By week 24, 57.0 % of the patients of the first group and 68.6 % of the patients of the second group reached NAPSI 75 on the target fingernail [64].

These studies prove that etanercept is an effective and safe treatment for nail psoriasis, but clinicians should inform patients that this modality is reacting probably slower than other biologics.

13.11.4.3 Adalimumab

Data from a prospective, open-label, uncontrolled study by van den Bosch et al., conducted in 9 European countries including 244 patients with psoriatic arthritis and nail dystrophy who concluded the 12-week period of treatment, suggest that adalimumab provided clinically important improvement in nail psoriasis in addition to joint and skin involvement utilizing total NAPSI score. An approximately 57 % decrease in the mean NAPSI score was demonstrated by week 12. In 103 patients, there was an optional extension period of treatment for 8 more weeks and the decrease of the mean NAPSI score was almost 91 % [65]. In a small cohort study, 7 patients with cutaneous and nail psoriasis and 14 patients with psoriatic arthritis and nail affection were treated with adalimumab 45 mg twice a month subcutaneously. Outcome measures were assessed at baseline and at weeks 12 and 24 using the NAPSI score. Six months later, in the patients of the first group, there was a decrease of NAPSI score by 85 % on the fingernail psoriasis and 71.5 % on the toenail psoriasis, and in the patients of the second group, respective numbers were 86 % for fingernails and 64 % for toenails. In this study an additional parameter which was investigated was the response on the Quality of Life Questionnaire which was filled by the patients. The initial burden on their quality of life of 61.10 ± 17.38 was reduced to 15,652 ± 8,453 at week 24 (69–83.5 %, mean 74 %) (Fig. 13.2a, b) [66]. Improvement in NAPSI score as high as 54 % at week 28 was reported in a randomized, placebo-controlled, double-blind trial study by Leonardi et al., where 36 patients were included [67].

13.11.4.4 Infliximab

Twenty-five patients with symptoms of nail psoriasis were treated with infliximab infusions at a dosage of 5 mg/kg, and at week 22 NAPSI-75 was achieved by all patients [68]. In a 50-week, phase III, randomized, double-blind trial in patients with moderate to severe psoriasis ($n = 373$), infliximab demonstrated efficacy with respect to improving nail psoriasis, as measured using NAPSI. The mean percentage of improvement in NAPSI from baseline to week 24 was 56.3 % [69]. In an unblinded, non-randomized, open-label study, 13 patients with psoriatic arthritis and 5 with severe plaque psoriasis and all with nail involvement were treated with infliximab infusions. NAPSI score was used to evaluate efficacy on nails and DLQI score to assess improvement in quality of life of these 18 patients. All 18 patients improved with a mean NAPSI score reduction from 55.78 before treatment to 3.28 at week 38 (almost complete clearance, 94 % improvement), while a significant reduction of the score of the international quality of life questionnaire was reported in all patients (from 66.28 to 19.11 at week 38, 75.5 % improvement) reflecting the satisfaction of patients from the improvement in the appearance of their nails (Fig. 13.3a, b) [70].

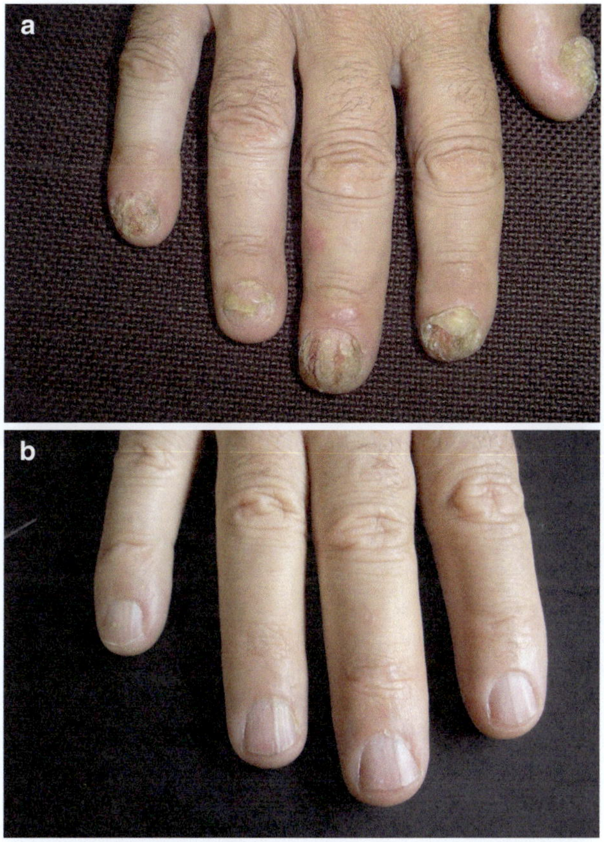

Fig. 13.2 (**a**) Adalimumab figure 1. (**b**) Adalimumab figure 2

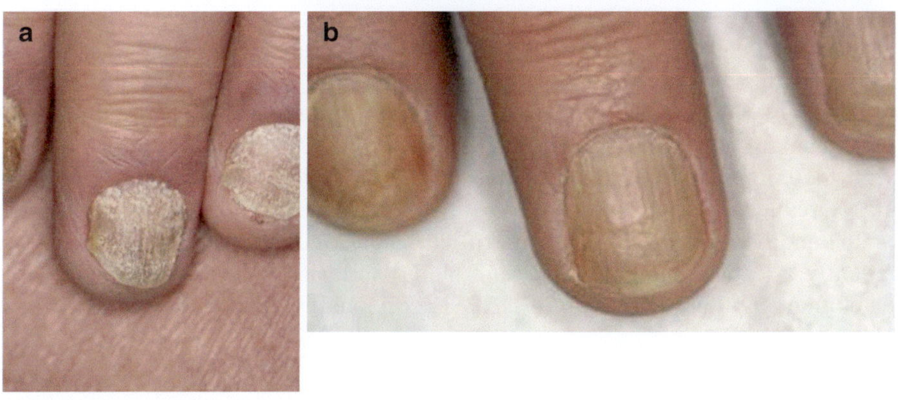

Fig. 13.3 (**a**) Infliximab before treatment. (**b**) Infliximab after treatment

In a randomized, double-blind, placebo-controlled multicenter study in Asian population, 28 patients with cutaneous psoriasis and psoriatic arthritis were treated with infliximab. According to the authors, the improvement in NAPSI score at week 10 was 1.4 ± 2.2 in the infliximab group compared with 0.3 ± 1.0 in the placebo group. NAPSI score improvement was further increased by 2.6 ± 2.0 at week 66 [71].

A rapid response consisting of almost 62.5 % improvement of NAPSI score at week 14, which increased further to 81 % at week 22 of infliximab treatment, was reported in an open-labeled study including 48 patients with nail psoriasis involvement (71 % of them has also psoriatic arthritis symptoms). At week 38, 29.2 % of the patients achieved NAPSI-90 score [72].

13.11.4.5 Ustekinumab

The anti-IL-12,-23 drug ustekinumab has also been studied in nail psoriasis, both in patients with and without psoriatic arthritis.

In one of the first published case reports, what is noticeable is the quick response of the patient with complete cure in 8 weeks that is just with two injections of the medication [73]. A mean 90 % reduction of NAPSI (from 19.8 on week 0 to 2.0 on week 40) and an 80 % improvement in QoL (from a score of 48.15 to a score of 10.0) in 40 weeks of treatment have been reported in an open prospective unblinded study which included 27 patients with cutaneous psoriasis and nail symptoms [74] (Fig. 13.4a, b). In 102 patients with nail psoriasis and moderate to severe skin disease, a double-blind, placebo-controlled study was conducted, and the authors conclude that in week 64 the mean percentage of improvement in target NAPSI was 56.6 ± 43.2 % and 67.8 ± 37.5 % for the 45 and 90 mg of ustekinumab, respectively. What is of interest in this study is that at week 12 improvement in NAPSI score of the target nails is low and not statistically significant compared to placebo [75].

Thirteen patients in total with skin psoriasis, psoriatic arthritis, and nail disease received treatment with ustekinumab according to their body weight (45 and 90 mg if the exceeded 90 kg). In eight patients that received the dosage of 45 mg, adjuvant treatment with 15–30 mg of MTX and in two with cyclosporine 200 mg/day was added. Five patients received 90 mg of ustekinumab as monotherapy. As the authors state, only NAPSI score for fingernails was used at week 12 to evaluate efficacy of treatment, as toenails grow slowly and at week 12 they cannot be assessed for any improvement. These 5 patients at week 12 presented with a reduction of NAPSI score of 37.6 %, the other 8 patients with the combination of ustekinumab 45 mg and MTX with a reduction of 27 %, and the last 2 patients with the combination of ustekinumab 45 mg and cyclosporine 200 mg, with a 100 % reduction of NAPSI score [76].

In another open-label, uncontrolled, non-randomized study published recently, 27 patients with skin and nail psoriasis received treatment with ustekinumab with a reduction of NAPSI score achieving 100 % after 40 weeks

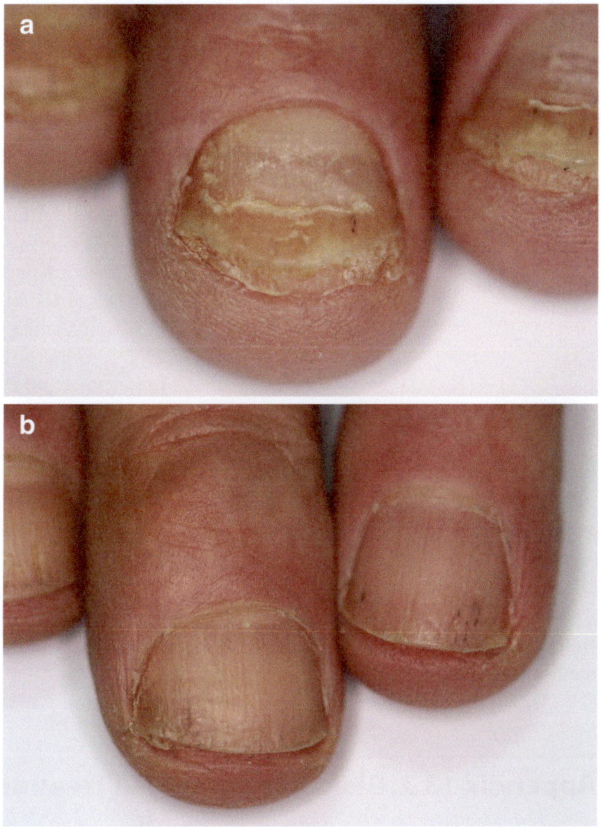

Fig. 13.4 (**a**) Patient 1, week 0 ustekinumab. (**b**) Patient 1, week 28 ustekinumab

of treatment. At week 16 a reduction of 49 % of the NAPSI score was noted, which was increased to almost 88 % at week 28, confirming the quick response that is noted on fingernail psoriasis with this medication [77]. In a large double-blind, randomized, placebo-controlled, multicenter trial, 545 psoriasis patients with fingernail disease were included and treated with ustekinumab according to the medication's protocol and the design of the study. NAPSI score, Nail Physician's Global Assessment (Nail PGA) and number of affected nails were the indexes for assessing drug's efficacy. NAPSI score was significantly improved from baseline to week 12 by 26.7 % in the 45 mg group and by 24.9 % in the 90 mg group of patients, signaling the early drug's efficacy. This improvement was increased at week 24 (46.5 and 48.7 %, respectively). Nail PGA was improved as expected at week 24, while a number of affected nails were improved already from week 12 [78].

So, in conclusion, all four existing biologic drugs seem to be effective in treating nail psoriasis with or without psoriatic arthritis symptoms.

Appendix 13.1. Traditional Systemic Medication (Only Studies Using NAPSI Score Are Included)

Name	Dosage	Efficacy
Acitretin	0.2–0.3 mg/kg/day	**41 % reduction of NAPSI after 24 weeks** [46]
	25 mg/day	18.5 % reduction of NAPSI after 12 weeks
		40.5 % reduction of NAPSI after 24 weeks
		51.7 % reduction of NAPSI after 48 weeks [49]
Cyclosporin A	3 mg/kg/day	37.8 % reduction of NAPSI after 12 weeks
		71.8 % reduction of NAPSI after 24 weeks
		89.1 % reduction of NAPSI after 48 weeks [49]
	5 mg/kg/day	**45.2 % reduction of NAPSI after 24 weeks for fingernails** and 37. 2 % reduction of NAPSI after 24 weeks for toenails [53]
Methotrexate	15 mg/week	**43.3 % reduction of NAPSI after 24 weeks** [54]
	15 mg/week	**36.8 % reduction of NAPSI after 24 weeks**
		39.3 % reduction of NAPSI after 52 weeks [55]
	7.5–25 mg/week	7.3 % reduction of NAPSI after 12 weeks
		30.8 % reduction of NAPSI after 24 weeks
		34. 9 % reduction of NAPSI after 48 weeks [49]
	15 mg/week	**49.3 % reduction of NAPSI after 24 weeks** [53]

Bold are used for numbers that are for the same period of treatment time, with different medication

Appendix 13.2. Biologics in the Nail Treatment

Name	Dosage	Efficacy
Etanercept	50 mg × 2/week ×12	76.1 % reduction in NAPSI score at week 24
	Afterwards, 50 mg × 1	92.8 % reduction in NAPSI score at week 48 [57]
	50 mg × 2/week	88.98 % achieved NAPSI 75 at week 36 [58]
	50 mg × 2/week	51 % reduction in NAPSI score at week 24 [63]
	50 mg × 2/week × 12 and afterwards 50 mg × once/week × 12	57 % reduction in NAPSI score at week 24
	OR	
	50 mg × 1/week × 24	68.6 % reduction in NAPSI score at week 24 [64]
Adalimumab	According to drug's protocol	70.2 % reduction in NAPSI score at week 24
	According to drug's protocol	89.5 % reduction in NAPSI score at week 48 [57]
	According to drug's protocol	93.75 % achieved NAPSI 75 at week 36 [58]
	According to drug's protocol	57 % reduction in NAPSI score at week 12 and 91 % in week 20 [65]
	According to drug's protocol	85 % reduction in NAPSI score at week 24 [66]
	According to drug's protocol	54 % reduction in NAPSI score at week 28 [67]

Name	Dosage	Efficacy
Infliximab	5 mg/kg	70.2 % reduction in NAPSI score at week 24
	5 mg/kg	95.1 % reduction in NAPSI score at week 48 [57]
	5 mg/kg	85.71 % achieved NAPSI 75 at week 36 [58]
	5 mg/kg	56.3 % reduction in NAPSI score at week 24 [69]
	5 mg/kg	94 % reduction in NAPSI score at week 38 [70]
	5 mg/kg	81 % reduction in NAPSI score at week 22 [72]
Ustekinumab	According to drug's protocol	83.33 % achieved NAPSI 75 at week 36 [58]
	According to drug's protocol	90 % reduction in NAPSI score at week 40 [74]
	According to drug's protocol	100 % reduction in NAPSI score at week 40 [77]
	According to drug's protocol	46.5 % reduction in NAPSI score at week 40 [78]

References

1. Oran Y, Akkaya D. Treatment of nail psoriasis: common concepts and new trends. Dermatol Res Pract. 2013;23:1–13.
2. Gregoriou S, Kalogeromitros D, Kosionis N, et al. Treatment options for nail psoriasis. Exp Rev Dermatol. 2008;3(3):339–44.
3. Radtke A, Beikert F, Augustin M. Nail psoriasis-a treatment challenge. J Dtsch Dermatol Ges. 2013;103:203–19.
4. Reich K. Approach to managing patients with nail psoriasis. J Eur Acad Dermatol Venereol. 2009;23 Suppl 1:15–21.
5. Jaravuthisan M, Sasseville D, Vender R, et al. Psoriasis of the nail: anatomy, pathology, clinical presentation, and a review of the literature on therapy. J Am Acad Dermatol. 2007;57:1–27.
6. Dehesa L, Tosti A. Treatment of inflammatory nail disorders. Dermatol Ther. 2012;25:525–34.
7. Cannavo SP, Guarneri F, Vaccaro M, et al. Treatment of psoriatic nails with topical cyclosporine: a prospective randomized, placebo-controlled study. Dermatology. 2003;206:153–6.
8. De Berker D, Lawrence CM. A simplified protocol of steroid injection for psoriatic nail dystrophy. Br J Dermatol. 1998;138:90–5.
9. De Berker D. Management of psoriatic nail disease. Semin Cutan Med Surg. 2009;28:39–43.
10. Saleem K, Azim W. Treatment of nail psoriasis with a modified regimen of steroid injections. J Coll Physicians Surg Pak. 2008;18(2):78–81.
11. De Berker D. Management of nail psoriasis. Clin Exp Dermatol. 2000;25:357–62.
12. Scher RK, Daniel CR. Nails: therapy, diagnosis, surgery. Philadelphia: W.B. Saunders Company; 2003.
13. Baran R, Tosti A. Treatment of nail psoriasis with a new corticoid –containing nail lacquer formulation. J Dermatol Treatm. 1999;10:201–4.
14. Sanchez Regana M, Martin Ezwuerra G, Millet U, et al. Treatment of nail psoriasis with 8 % clobetasol nail lacquer: positive experience in 10 patients. J Eur Acad Dermatol Venereol. 2005;19:573–7.
15. Nakamura R, Duque-Estrada B, Pizzaro Leverone A, et al. Comparison of nail lacquer clobetasol efficacy at 0, 05 %, 1 % and 8 % in nail psoriasis treatment: prospective, controlled and randomized pilot study. An Bras Dermatol. 2012;87(2):203–11.
16. van Le Q, Howard A. Dexamethasone iontophoresis for the treatment of nail psoriasis. Aust J Dermatol. 2013;54:115–9.

17. Tosti A, Piraccini BM, Cameli N, et al. Calcipotriol ointment in nail psoriasis: a controlled, double-blind comparison with betamethasone dipropionate and salicylic acid. Br J Dermatol. 1998;139:655–9.
18. Zakeri M, Valikhani M, Mortazavi H, et al. Topical calcipotriol therapy in nail psoriasis: a study of 24 cases. Dermatol Online J. 2005;11(3):5–9.
19. Rigopoulos D, Ioannides D, Prastitis N, et al. Nail psoriasis: a combined treatment using calcipotriol cream and clobetasol propionate cream. Acta Dermatol Venereol. 2002;82(2):140–3.
20. Piraccini BM, Tosti A, Iorizzo M, et al. Pustular psoriasis of the nails: treatment and long-term follow-up of 46 patients. Br J Dermatol. 2001;144:1000–5.
21. Balbas-Marquez M, Sanchez-Regana M, Millet-Umbert P. Tacalcitol ointment for the treatment of nail psoriasis. J Dermatol Treat. 2009;20(5):308–10.
22. Scher RK, Stiller M, Zhu YI. Tazarotene 0.1 % gel in the treatment of fingernail psoriasis: a double-blind, randomized, vehicle-controlled study. Cutis. 2001;68:355–8.
23. Bianchi L, Soda R, Diluvio L, et al. Tazarotene 0.1 % gel for psoriasis of the fingernails and toenails: an open, prospective study. Br J Dermatol. 2003;149(1):207–9.
24. Rigopoulos D, Gregoriou S, Katsambas A. Treatment of psoriatic nails with Tazarotene 0.1 % gel vs clobetasol propionate 0.05 % cream: a double-blind study. Acta Derm Venereol. 2007;87(2):167–8.
25. Levancini-Fischer C, Sanchez-Regana M, Lambi F, et al. Nail psoriasis: treatment with Tazarotene 0.1 % hydrophilic ointment. Actas Dermosifiliogr. 2012;103(8):725–8.
26. Fredricksson T. Topically applied fluorouracil in the treatment of psoriatic nails. Arch Dermatol. 1974;110:735–6.
27. Fritz K. Successful local treatment of nail psoriasis with 5-fluorouracil. Z Hautkr. 1989; 15(64):1083–8.
28. de Jong EM, Menke HE, van Praag MC, et al. Dystrophic psoriatic fingernails treated with 1 % fluorouracil in a nail-penetration-enhancing vehicle. Dermatology. 1999;199:313–8.
29. Yamamoto T, Katayana I, Nishioka K. Topical anthralin therapy for refractory nail psoriasis. J Dermatol. 1998;25(4):231–3.
30. De Simone C, Maiorino A, Tassone F, et al. Tacrolimus 0,1 % ointment in nail psoriasis: a randomized, controlled, open-label study. J Eur Acad Dermatol Venereol. 2013;27:1003–6.
31. Hoffmann C, Plewig G. Photochemotherapie der nagelpsoriasis. Hautarzt. 1977;28:498–9.
32. Handfield-Jones SE, Boyle J, Harman RRM. Local PUVA treatment for nail psoriasis. Br J Dermatol. 1987;116(2):280–1.
33. Stern DK, Creasey AA, Quigigie J, et al. UVA and UVB penetration of normal human cadaveric fingernail plate. Arch Dermatol. 2011;147(4):439–41.
34. Trieewittayapoon C, Sigvahamont P, Chanprapaph K, et al. The effect of different pulse durations in the treatment of nail psoriasis with 595-nm pulsed dye laser: a randomized, double-blind, intrapatient left-to-right study. J Am Acd Dermatol. 2012;66:807–12.
35. Oram Y, Karincaoğlu Y, Koyuncu E, et al. Pulsed dye laser in the treatment of nail psoriasis. Dermatol Surg. 2010;36(3):377–81.
36. Al-Mutairi A, Elkashlan M. Nail psoriasis treated with pulse dye laser. Indian J Dermatol. 2013;58(3):243–5.
37. Fernández-Guarino M, Harto A, Sánchez-Ronco M, et al. Pulsed dye laser vs photodynamic therapy in the treatment of refractory nail psoriasis: a comparative pilot study. J Eur Acad Dermatol Venereol. 2009;23(8):891–5.
38. Rigopoulos D, Gregoriou S, Daniel CR, et al. Treatment of nail psoriasis with a two compound formulation of calcipotriol plus betamethasone dipropionate ointment. Dermatology. 2009;218:338–41.
39. Sanchez Regana M, Marquez Balbas G, Millet Umbert P. Nail psoriasis: a combined treatment with 8 % clobetasol nail laquer and tacalcitol ointment. J Eur Acad Dermatol Venereol. 2008;22:963–9.
40. Huang YC, Chou CL, Chiang YY. Efficacy of pulsed dye laser plus topical tazarotene versus topical tazarotene alone in psoriatic nail disease: a single-blind, intrapatient left-to-right controlled study. Lasers Surg Med. 2013;45(2):102–7.

41. Cantoresi F, Sorgi P, Arcese A, et al. Improvement of psoriatic onychodystrophy by a water-soluble nail lacquer. J Eur Acad Dermatol Venereol. 2009;23:832–4.
42. Vlachou C, Berth-Jones J. Nail psoriasis improvement in a patient treated with fumaric acid esters. J Dermatol Treat. 2007;18:175–7.
43. Lindelof B. Psoriasis of the nails treated with grenz rays: a double-blind bilateral trial. Acta Derm Venereol. 1989;69(1):80–2.
44. Yu RC, King CM. A double-blind study of superficial radiotherapy in psoriatic nail dystrophy. Acta Derm Venereol. 1992;72(2):134–6.
45. Kwang TY, Nee TS, Seng KT. A therapeutic study of nail psoriasis using electron beam. Acta Derm Venereol. 1995;75(1):90–2.
46. Tosti A, Ricotti C, Romanelli P, et al. Evaluation of the efficacy of Acitretin therapy for nail psoriasis. Arch Dermatol. 2009;145(3):269–71.
47. Ricceri F, Pescitelli L, Tripo L, et al. Treatment of severe nail psoriasis with psoriasis: an impressive therapeutic result. Dermatol Ther. 2013;26(1):77–8.
48. Mahrle G, Schultze HG, Farber L, et al. Low- dose short-term cyclosporine versus etretinate in psoriasis: improvement of skin, nails and joint involvement. J Am Acad Dermatol. 1995;32:78–88.
49. Sanchez-Regana M, Sola-Ortigosa J, Gibert-Alsina J, et al. Nail psoriasis: a retrospective study on the effectiveness of systemic treatment (classical and biological therapy). J Eur Acad Dermatol Venereol. 2011;25:57–586.
50. Ojeda R, Sanchez-Regana M, Massana J, et al. Clinical experience with the use of cyclosporine A in psoriasis, Results of a retrospective study. J Dermatol Treat. 2005;16:338–41.
51. Feliciani C, Zampetti A, Forleo P, et al. Nail psoriasis: combined therapy with systemic cyclosporine and topical calcipotriol. J Cutan Med Surg. 2004;8:122–5.
52. Syuto T, Abe M, Ishibuchi H, et al. Successful treatment of psoriatic nails with low-dose cyclosporine administration. Eur J Dermatol. 2007;17(3):248–9.
53. Gumusel M, Ozdemir M, Mevlitoglou I, et al. Evaluation of the efficacy of methotrexate and cyclosporine therapies on psoriatic nails: a one-blind, randomized study. J Eur Acad Dermatol Venereol. 2011;25:1080–4.
54. Lee JY. Severe 20-nail psoriasis successfully treated by low dose methotrexate. Dermatol Online. 2009;15(11):8–11.
55. Reich N, Nestle FO, Papp K, et al. Infliximab induction and maintenance therapy for moderate-to-severe psoriasis: a phase III multicentre double-blind trial. Lancet. 2005;366:1367–74.
56. Saricaoglu H, Oz A, Turan H. Nail psoriasis successfully treated with intralesional methotrexate: case report. Dermatology. 2011;222(1):5–7.
57. Kyriakou A, Patsatsi A, Sotiriadis D. Anti-TNF agents and nail psoriasis: a single-center, retrospective, comparative study. J Dermatol Treat. 2013;24(3):162–8.
58. Bardazzi F, Antonucci V, Odorici G, et al. A 36-week retrospective open trial comparing the efficacy of biological therapies in nail psoriasis. J Dtsch Dermatol Ges. 2013;11:1065–70.
59. Cassetty CT, Alexis AF, Shupack JL, et al. Alefacept in the treatment of psoriatic nail disease: a small case series. J Am Acad Dermatol. 2005;52(6):1101–2.
60. Körver JE, Langewouters AM, Van De Kerkhof PC, et al. Therapeutic effects of a 12-week course of Alefacept on nail psoriasis. J Eur Acad Dermatol Venereol. 2006;20(10):1252–5.
61. Parrish CA, Sobera JO, Robbins CM, et al. Alefacept in the treatment of psoriatic nail disease: a proof of concept study. J Drugs Dermatol. 2006;5(4):339–40.
62. Oram Y, Akkaya D. Treatment of nail psoriasis: common concepts and new trends. Dermatol Res Pract. 2013;2013:180496.
63. Luger TA, Barker J, Lambert J, et al. Sustained improvement in joint pain and nail symptoms with Etanercept therapy in patients with moderate-to-severe psoriasis. J Eur Acad Dermatol Venereol. 2009;23(8):896–904.
64. Ortonne JP, Paul C, Berardesca E, et al. A 24-week randomized clinical trial investigating the efficacy and safety of two doses of Etanercept in nail psoriasis. Br J Dermatol. 2013;168(5):1080–7.
65. Van den Bosch F, Manger B, Goupille P, et al. Effectiveness of Adalimumab in treating patients with active psoriatic arthritis and predictors of good clinical responses for arthritis, skin and nail lesions. Ann Rheum Dis. 2010;69(2):394–9.

66. Rigopoulos D, Gregoriou S, Lazaridou E, et al. Treatment of nail psoriasis with Adalimumab. An open label, uncontrolled study. J Eur Acad Dermatol Venereol. 2010;24(5):530–4.
67. Leonardi C, Langley RG, Papp K, et al. Adalimumab for the treatment of moderate to severe chronic plaque psoriasis of the hands and feet: efficacy and safety results from REACH a randomized, placebo-controlled, double-blind trial. Arch Dermatol. 2011;147(4):429–36.
68. Bianchi L, Bergamin A, de Felice C, et al. Remission and time of resolution of nail psoriasis during Infliximab therapy. J Am Acad Dermatol. 2005;52(4):736–7.
69. Rich P, Griffiths C, Reich K, et al. Baseline nail disease in patients with moderate to severe psoriasis and response to treatment with Infliximab during 1 year. J Am Acad Dermatol. 2008;58:224–31.
70. Rigopoulos D, Gregoriou S, Stratigos A, et al. Evaluation of the efficacy and safety of Infliximab on psoriatic nails: an unblinded, non-randomized, open-label study. Br J Dermatol. 2008;159(2):453–6.
71. Torii H, Nakagawa H. Infliximab monotherapy in Japanese patients with moderate-to-severe plaque psoriasis and psoriatic arthritis. A randomized, double-blind, placebo-controlled multicenter trial. J Dermatol Sci. 2010;59:40–9.
72. Fabroni C, Gori A, Troiano M, et al. Infliximab efficacy in nail psoriasis. A retrospective study in 48 patients. J Eur Acad Dermatol Venereol. 2011;25:549–63.
73. Rallis E, Kintzoglou S, Verros C. Ustekinumab for rapid treatment of nail psoriasis. Arch Dermatol. 2010;146:1315–6.
74. Rigopoulos D, Gregoriou S, Makris M, et al. Efficacy of ustekinumab in nail psoriasis and improvement in nail-associated quality of life in a population treated with ustekinumab for cutaneous psoriasis: an open prospective unblinded study. Dermatology. 2011;223:325–9.
75. Igarashi A, Kato T, Kato M, et al. Efficacy and safety of ustekinumab in Japanese patients with moderate-to-severe plaque-type psoriasis: long-term results from a phase 2/3 clinical trial. J Dermatol. 2012;39:242–52.
76. Vitiello M, Tosti A, Abuchar A, et al. Ustekinumab for the treatment of nail psoriasis in heavily treated psoriatic patients. Int J Dermatol. 2013;52:358–62.
77. Patsatsi A, Kyriakou A, Sotiriadis D. Ustekinumab in nail psoriasis: an open-label, uncontrolled, nonrandomized study. J Dermatolog Treat. 2013;24:96–100.
78. Rich P, Bourcier M, Sofen H, et al. Ustekinumab improves nail disease in patients with moderate to-severe psoriasis: results from PHOENIX 1. Br J Dermatol. 2014;170(2):398–407.

Nail Psoriasis in Special Populations: Children, Pregnant, Elderly

14

Bianca Maria Piraccini and Michela Starace

Contents

Key Features

- Nail psoriasis in children is rare and usually mild.
- Frequency and severity of nail psoriasis do not change in pregnancy.
- Onset of nail psoriasis in the elderly is very rare.
- Hallopeau's acrodermatitis continua is the most common variety of nail psoriasis in adulthood and old age.
- Pustular psoriasis of the nails in children is extremely infrequent.

B.M. Piraccini, MD, PhD (✉) • M. Starace, MD
Division of Dermatology, Department of Specialized, Experimental and Diagnostic Medicine, University of Bologna, Bologna, Italy
e-mail: biancamaria.piraccini@unibo.it; michela.starace2@unibo.it

D. Rigopoulos, A. Tosti (eds.), *Nail Psoriasis: From A to Z*,
DOI 10.1007/978-3-319-08810-5_14

14.1 Introduction

Nail psoriasis can occur at any age, associated or not to skin and/or arthropathic psoriasis.

The frequency, severity, and association of nail psoriasis with skin and/or joint psoriasis are different in the different age groups, as it is the approach to the disease, since choice of therapy is quite difficult in both age groups.

This chapter will review nail psoriasis in children and elderly (people older than 60 years), using the data found in the literature and my two-decade personal experience in an outpatient consultation for nail diseases.

14.2 Epidemiology

Nail psoriasis is reported to occur in up to 40 % of children who suffer from skin psoriasis, with figures that do not significantly differ worldwide [1–8]. Involvement of the nails has no relationship with type of psoriasis or duration or extent of disease. Besides two studies [4, 8], reporting a higher frequency of nail changes in boys than in girls with skin psoriasis, no gender predilection is generally found. Differently from adults, in children nail involvement does not correlate with psoriatic arthritis. Age of appearance of nail lesions is around 7–12 years.

There are no epidemiological data on the frequency of psoriasis limited to the nails in children. It is not rare, but it possibly goes unnoticed by the child and the parents, as a mild pitting or toenail thickening, the most common signs, are often considered not worrisome and in need of a specialist consultation.

Skin psoriasis may occur in persons over 60 years old (elderly-onset psoriasis), and the frequency of nail involvement does not seem different in that age compared to that of younger psoriatic patients [9]. Isolated nail psoriasis may occur in the elderly, and the acral variety of pustular psoriasis (Hallopeau's acrodermatitis continua) is typical of adult-elderly persons [10].

14.3 Clinical Features

Clinical features are shown in Table 14.1.

Nail psoriasis in children: nail symptoms are usually mild and frequently go unnoticed by the child and the parents.

- In the fingernails, psoriasis in children typically produces a mild *pitting*. Pitting results from psoriatic involvement of the proximal nail matrix with focal defective keratinization of nail matrix cells and persistence of groups of nucleated and incompletely keratinized (parakeratotic) cells on the nail plate surface. These cells poorly adhere to each other and detach to the nail plate surface leaving small holes, the pits, which appear as punctate depressions (Fig. 14.1). Pitting is rarely seen in the toenails (Fig. 14.2) and it is not exclusive of psoriasis, as it can

Table 14.1 Clinical features of nail psoriasis in special populations

Nail psoriasis in children
In up to 40 % of children with skin psoriasis
Isolated nail lesions rare
Age of onset 7–12 years
Usually mild
Fingernails: pitting
Toenails: nail plate thickening
Pustular psoriasis exceptional
Nail psoriasis in the elderly
No data about prevalence of nail involvement in elderly-onset skin psoriasis
Isolated nail lesions rare
Hallopeau's acrodermatitis typical of this age group

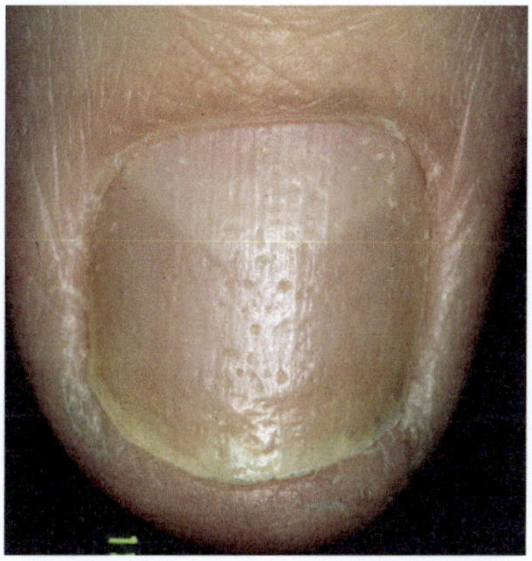

Fig. 14.1 Pitting, punctate depressions of the nail plate, is the most frequent sign of nail psoriasis in children

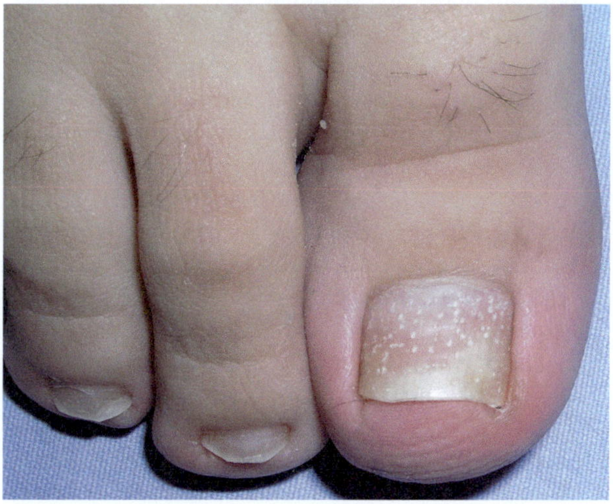

Fig. 14.2 Toenail pitting in a 13-year-old girl. Psoriatic pits are filled by scales

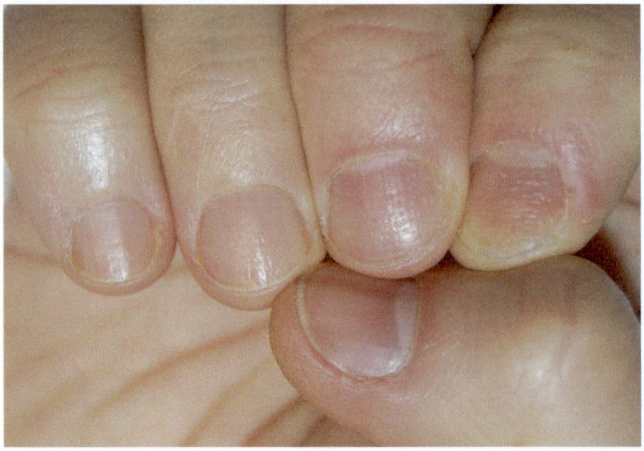

Fig. 14.3 Nail psoriasis in a 9-year-old boy. The severity varies from nail to nail

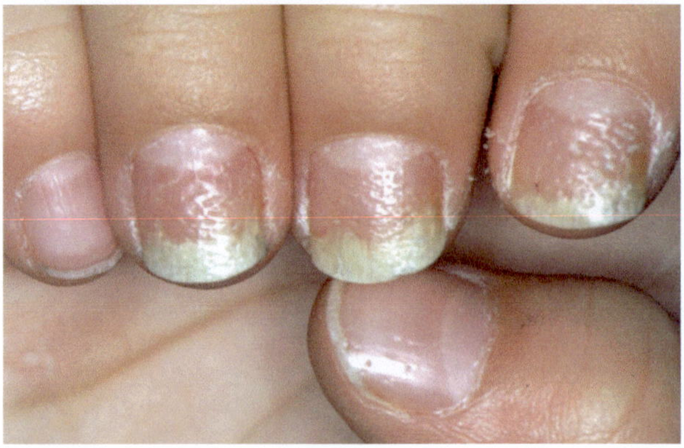

Fig. 14.4 Nail psoriasis in an 8-year-old girl: pitting is severe and involves several nails

be also seen in alopecia areata of the nails and in eczema. Psoriatic pits are typically large and irregular in shape and distribution (Fig. 14.3). In children, pitting is usually mild and limited to one or to a few digits, and it is only rarely associated to other signs of nail psoriasis (Fig. 14.3). Involvement of several digits with evident nail dystrophy is uncommon (Fig. 14.4).

- The second most common sign of nail psoriasis in children is *onycholysis associated with subungual hyperkeratosis*. The term onycholysis describes detachment of the nail plate from the underlying nail bed. The nail plate appears white due to the presence of air underneath it. Subungual hyperkeratosis results from excessive proliferation of nail bed/hyponychium keratinocytes that leads to accumulation of scales under the nail plate. Onycholysis and subungual hyperkeratosis are often present together in childhood nail psoriasis and may be seen in the fingernails (Fig. 14.5), but are more frequently evident in the toenails (Fig. 14.6). They typically involve several nails, not necessarily of the great toes. This is an important diagnostic clue. Splinter hemorrhages may be associated, favored by trauma. The salmon-pink erythematous border (oil drop sign) that in psoriasis usually surrounds the onycholytic area may be absent or scarcely

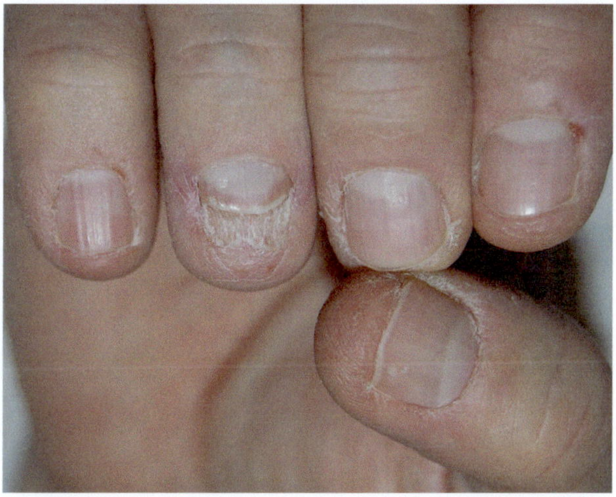

Fig. 14.5 Nail psoriasis in a 12-year-old girl: the fourth fingernail shows onycholysis and mild subungual hyperkeratosis

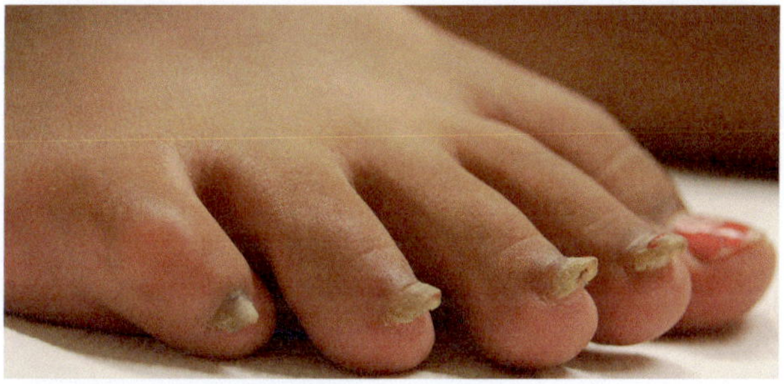

Fig. 14.6 Nail psoriasis in a 9-year-old girl: several toenails show onycholysis and subungual hyperkeratosis

visible in children's toenails (Fig. 14.7), making diagnosis difficult in the absence of skin signs of psoriasis. As trauma worsens nail symptoms, nail biting worsens onycholysis and subungual hyperkeratosis in fingernail psoriasis (Fig. 14.8). Differential diagnosis involves other diseases that cause onycholysis and subungual hyperkeratosis, mainly distal subungual onychomycosis and eczema. Onychomycosis is rare in children, where it can be limited to a single digit, including the fingernails [11]. The nail signs may be clinically indistinguishable from those of nail psoriasis, and differential diagnosis can be impossible without mycology (Fig. 14.9). Eczema in childhood is commonly due to atopic dermatitis, which can involve the hand and the periungual tissues, causing mild onycholysis and subungual hyperkeratosis (Fig. 14.10). Nail signs are always associated with dermatitis of the dorsal of the volar skin of the hand. Nail thickening with increased transverse curvature due to severe nail bed hyperkeratosis with onset in childhood is a typical finding of pachyonychia congenital, where they involve all 20 nails with different degrees of severity [12]. The family history and the associated findings lead to the diagnosis.

- *Nail plate thickening* with difficult nail trimming, involving several toenails, is in my experience a common sign of presentation of nail psoriasis at very young

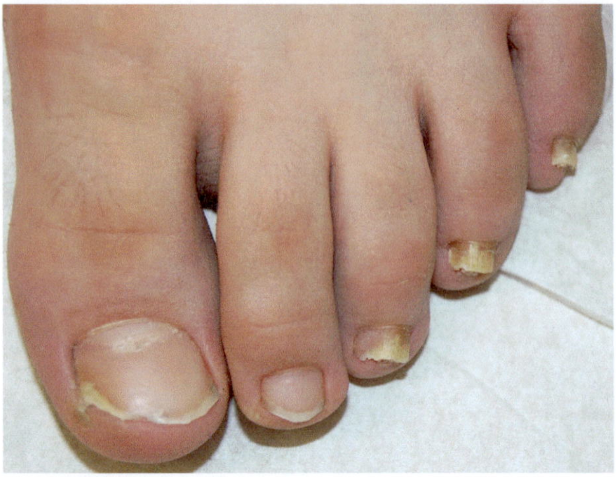

Fig. 14.7 Nail psoriasis in an 11-year-old boy. Only some toenails are affected with onycholysis and subungual hyperkeratosis causing nail thickening. The erythematous border that limits the onycholysis is scarcely evident

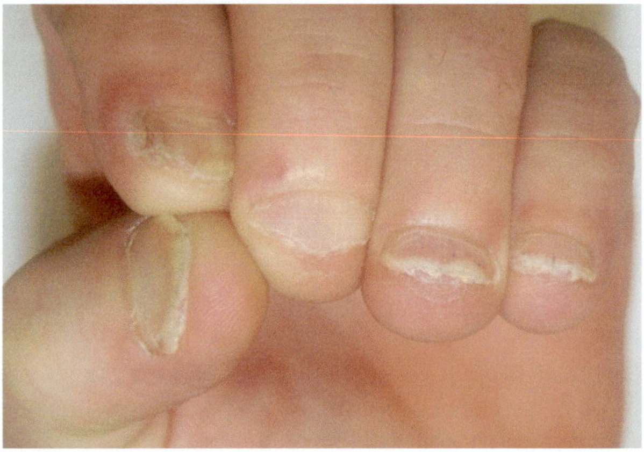

Fig. 14.8 Nail psoriasis in a 14-year-old boy with the habit of nail biting. The nails are short due to biting, and they show onycholysis, subungual hyperkeratosis, and splinter hemorrhages worsened by the mechanical trauma

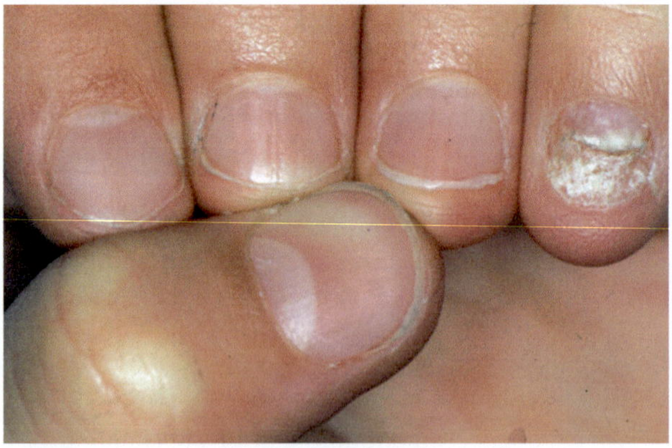

Fig. 14.9 Onychomycosis due to *Trichophyton rubrum* of the fifth fingernail in a 7-year-old girl: onycholysis and subungual hyperkeratosis strongly resemble those due to nail psoriasis

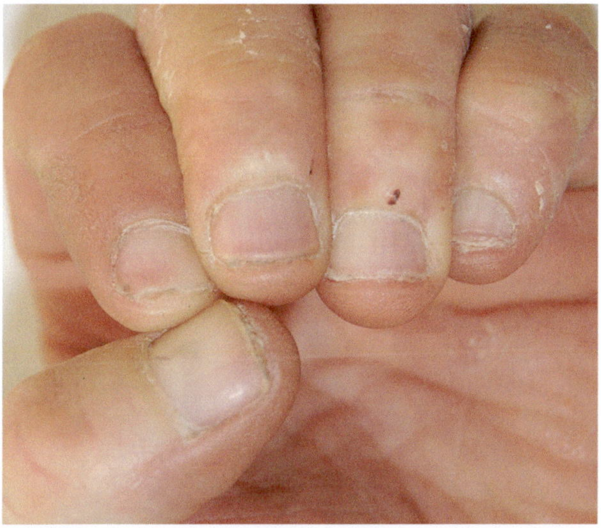

Fig. 14.10 Atopic eczema in a 10-year-old boy. Skin signs of chronic dermatitis are associated with mild onycholysis and subungual hyperkeratosis

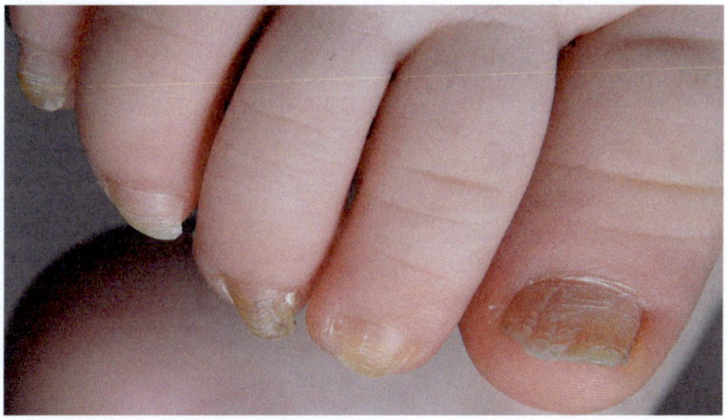

Fig. 14.11 Nail psoriasis in a 2-year-old boy: nail thickening with difficult nail trimming is the most evident sign

age: the parents notice gradual thickening of one of several nail plates of the child's toenails that are difficult to trim (Fig. 14.11). Differential diagnosis includes onychogryphosis, which is rare in children, especially below the age of 10 years, and usually involves the 1st toenail.

- *Parakeratosis pustulosa* is a possible clinical variety of nail psoriasis in children [13]. It is usually limited to one digit, most often the thumb or the index finger, which shows mild psoriasiform changes more marked on one side of the nail (Fig. 14.12). In most patients, nail signs are associated or preceded by erythema, scaling, and vesicles of the fingertip. Differential diagnosis includes eczema, and patch tests may show allergic contact dermatitis. Parakeratosis pustulosa either regresses spontaneously or evolves in nail psoriasis.
- Nail psoriasis may also appear as *trachyonychia*. Trachyonychia, or twenty-nail dystrophy, is an acquired benign inflammation of the proximal nail matrix that produces characteristic nail plate surface abnormalities [14]. The affected nail shows diffuse homogeneous roughness, due to fine superficial striations

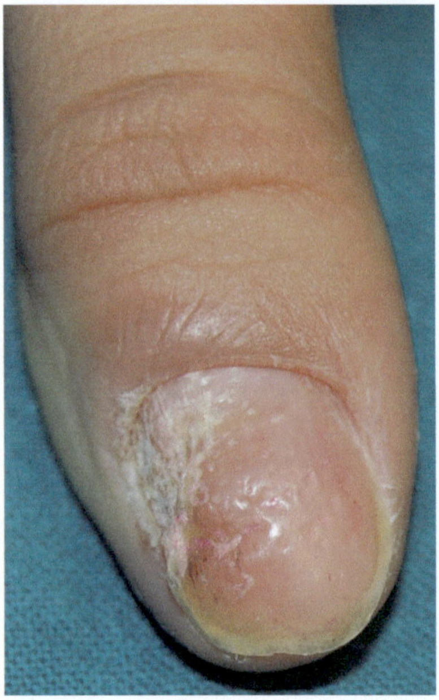

Fig. 14.12 Parakeratosis pustulosa in a 13-year-old girl: one fingernail shows pitting, nail plate surface abnormalities, and salmon-pink discoloration, which are more marked on one side of the nail

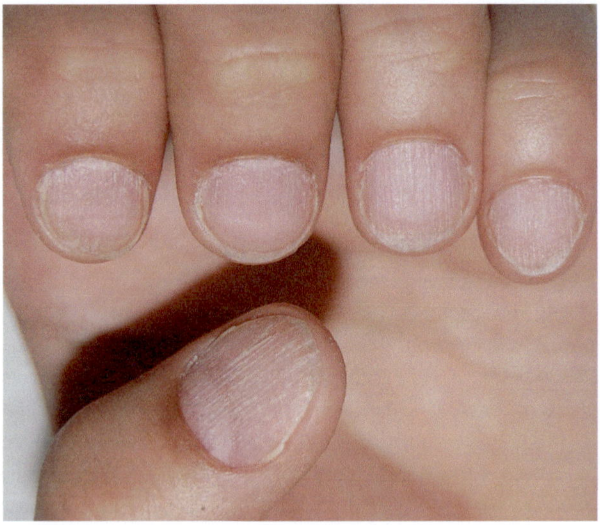

Fig. 14.13 Trachyonychia in an 8-year-old girl. The nails are rough, due to multiple regular superficial longitudinal striations

distributed in a regular, longitudinal, parallel pattern (Fig. 14.13). Small, superficial, adherent scales may be present. Nail thinning with koilonychia is frequent, as well as hyperkeratosis of the cuticles (Fig. 14.14). Trachyonychia may affect one, several, or all nails and can be due to different inflammatory diseases, such as alopecia areata, psoriasis, eczema, and lichen planus. In the

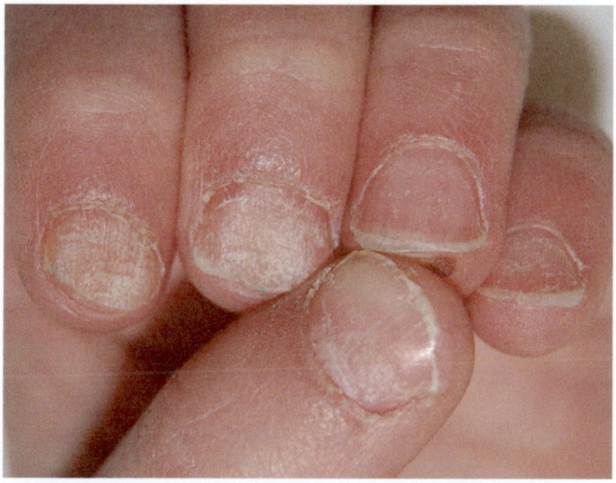

Fig. 14.14 Trachyonychia in a 7-year-old boy. Severity of nail signs varies in the different nails, with the second and third fingernails showing the more severe changes: nail roughness due to longitudinal striations is associated with thinning and koilonychia. Note mild hyperkeratosis of the cuticles

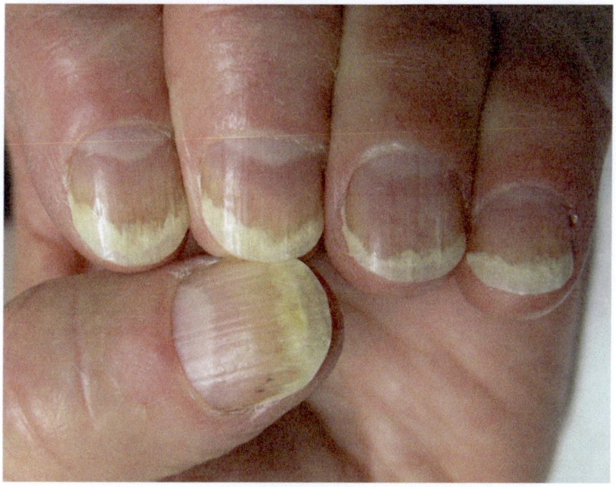

Fig. 14.15 Nail psoriasis with typical signs in a 72-year-old woman: the fingernails show onycholysis with erythematous border and some splinter hemorrhages

absence of anamnestic or clinical data that suggest the pathology, it is impossible to detect the disease that is causing trachyonychia without a histopathological study. A nail biopsy is however not indicated in trachyonychia, as it is usually a benign condition that tends to improve with time.

Nail psoriasis in the elderly: nail signs are similar to those seen in adults with nail psoriasis.

- The most common clinical presentation of nail psoriasis in the elderly is *onycholysis with erythematous border*, which can affect the fingernails (Fig. 14.15) and the toenails (Fig. 14.16), together or separately. When the toenails are the exclusive site of involvement, differential diagnosis with traumatic onycholysis and distal subungual onychomycosis is very difficult (Fig. 14.17). Dermoscopy may be helpful, as it visualizes the salmon-pink border surrounding the distal

Fig. 14.16 Same patient of Fig. 14.15: psoriasis produces onycholysis with erythematous border of the great toenail

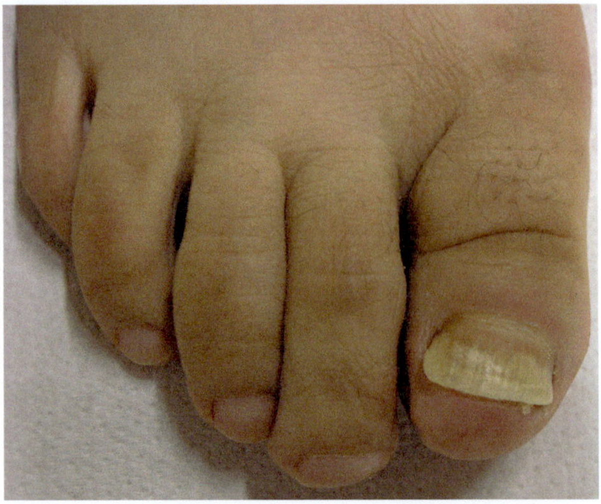

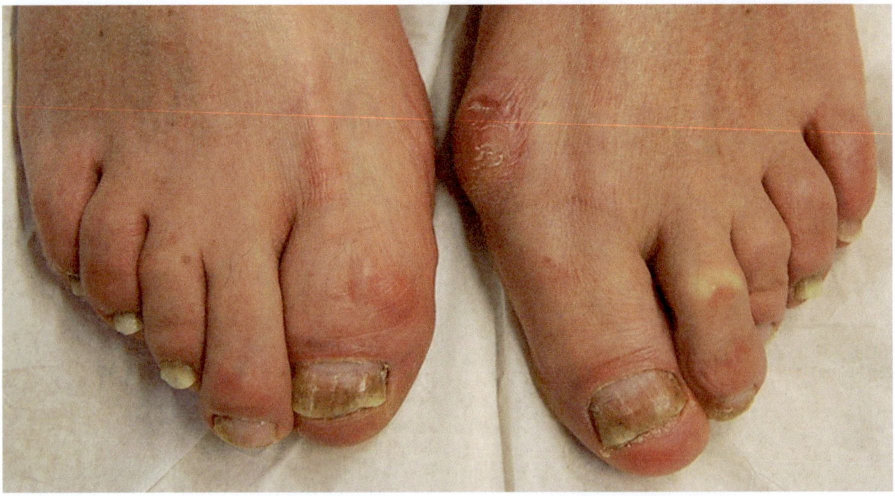

Fig. 14.17 Psoriasis limited to the toenails in a 78-year-old man without any skin lesion. Onycholysis, subungual hyperkeratosis, and splinter hemorrhages are not specific and do not allow differentiation from onychomycosis

detachment and the associated splinter hemorrhages (Fig. 14.18) [15], and does not show the typical features of onychomycosis [16], but mycology is always required to rule out onychomycosis. In our experience, nail psoriasis does not predispose to onychomycosis.

- Nail psoriasis in the elderly may sometimes affect one or a few fingernails and induce only *nail plate surface abnormalities* (Figs. 14.19 and 14.20). Differential diagnosis is again with fingernail onychomycosis, which may present in the same way. Examination of the 20 nails, the palms, and the soles, together with mycology, is necessary in these cases.

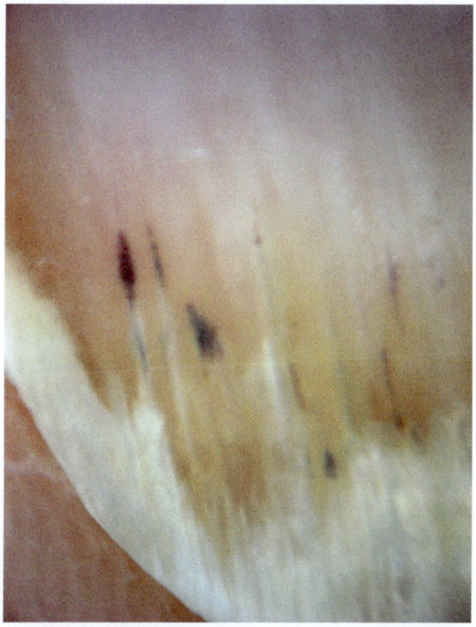

Fig. 14.18 Dermoscopy of nail psoriasis showing the pink-yellow border that surrounds the onycholysis and better visualize splinter hemorrhages. The technique helps in differential diagnosis with distal subungual onychomycosis, but does not substitute mycology

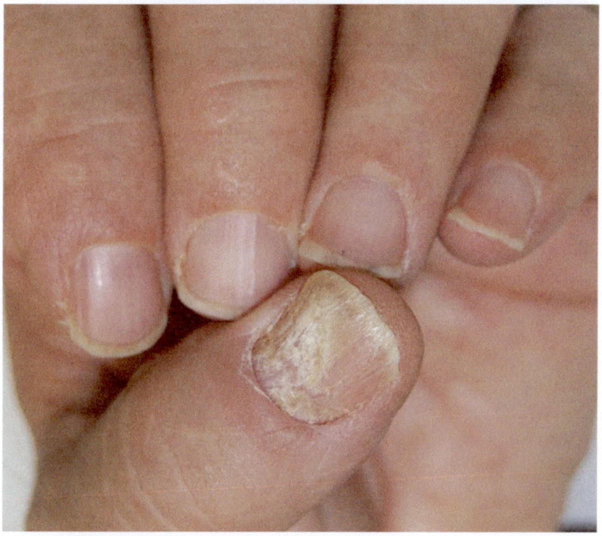

Fig. 14.19 Nail psoriasis in a 66-year-old man. Exclusive involvement of the nail matrix of the first finger produces nail plate surface abnormalities

- Pustular psoriasis of the nails may have onset in old age, both in the variant palmoplantar pustular psoriasis and as Hallopeau's acrodermatitis continua. *Palmoplantar pustular psoriasis* with nail involvement is characterized by acute inflammation with pustules involving the palmoplantar skin, the periungual tissues (Fig. 14.21), and the nail bed, with nail plate destruction, erosions, and crusts (Figs. 14.21, 14.22, and 14.23). Pain is a common complain. *Hallopeau's acrodermatitis continua* is a chronic-recurrent variant of pustular psoriasis that

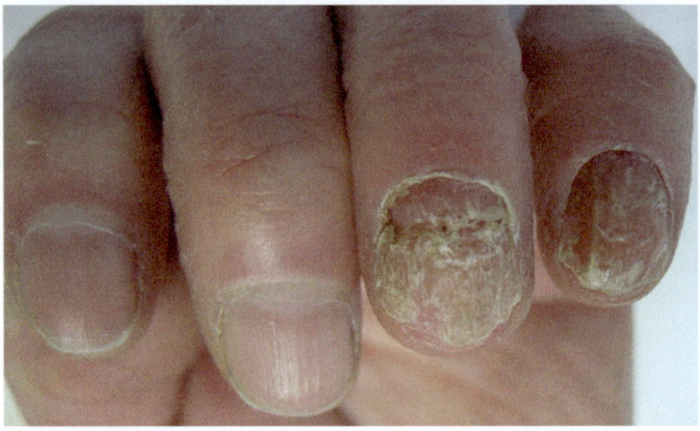

Fig. 14.20 Nail psoriasis in a 67-year-old woman. The fourth and fifth fingernails show surface abnormalities that resemble those due to onychomycosis of the fingernails

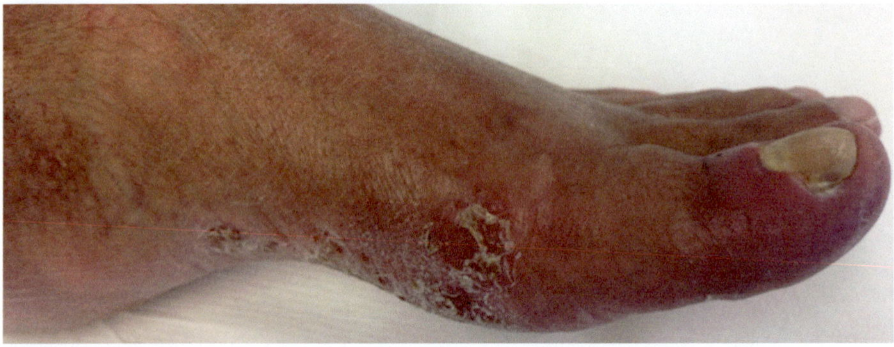

Fig. 14.21 Palmoplantar pustular psoriasis in a 66-year-old man. The plantar skin shows inflammation with pustules and crusts and the periungual skin of the great toe is markedly inflamed, with pustules under the nail plate

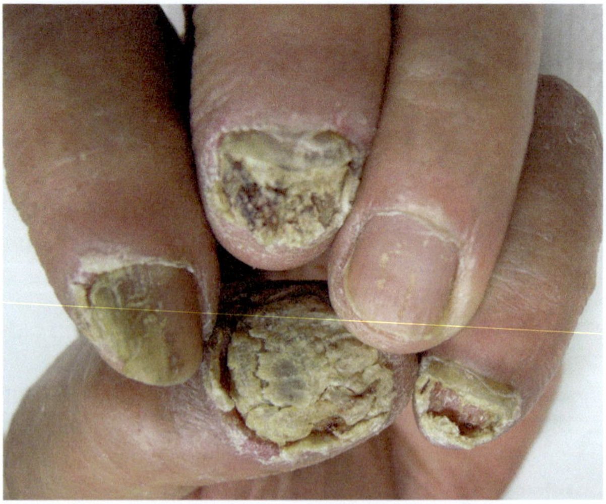

Fig. 14.22 Palmoplantar pustular psoriasis in a 64-year-old man: the nail bed is the site of the pathology with onycholysis, erosions, and thick crusts. Note psoriasiform lesions of the proximal nail folds

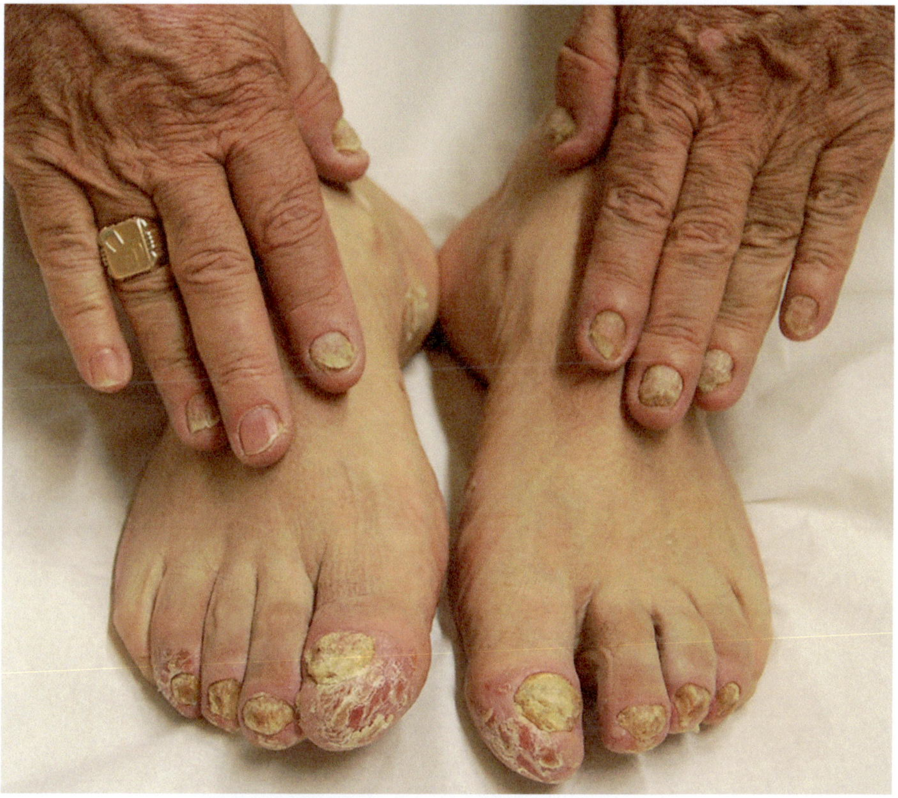

Fig. 14.23 Palmoplantar pustular psoriasis in a 70-year-old man. The lesions involve the skin and the nails of the hands and feet, with signs more severe in the toenails

has a typical onset in adulthood and old age [10] and involves the distal part of one or a few digits, including the nails. In acute phase, the affected digits show periungual and subungual pustules with onycholysis or nail plate destruction (Figs. 14.24 and 14.25). When the acute episode has subsided, the affected digit shows onycholysis with periungual erythema and nail bed scaling (Fig. 14.26). Pustular psoriasis may destroy the nail apparatus causing definitive loss of the nail. Acro-osteolysis due to bone resorption is fortunately uncommon [17] (Figs. 14.27 and 14.28).

14.4 Diagnostic Clues

- Look at all the 20 nails in order not to miss onychodystrophies that the parents, or the old patient, have not noticed.
- Look at the symptoms of the affected nails and detect the site of the nail apparatus that is affected: nail matrix, nail bed, and proximal nail fold.

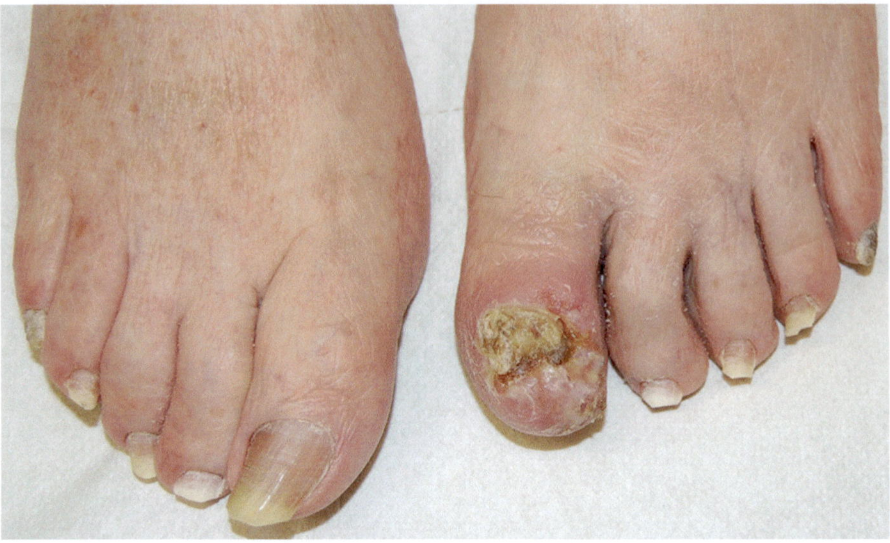

Fig. 14.24 Hallopeau's acrodermatitis continua in a 77-year-old woman. The left great toenail shows acute periungual inflammation with nail plate absence and pustules of the nail bed and distal pulp

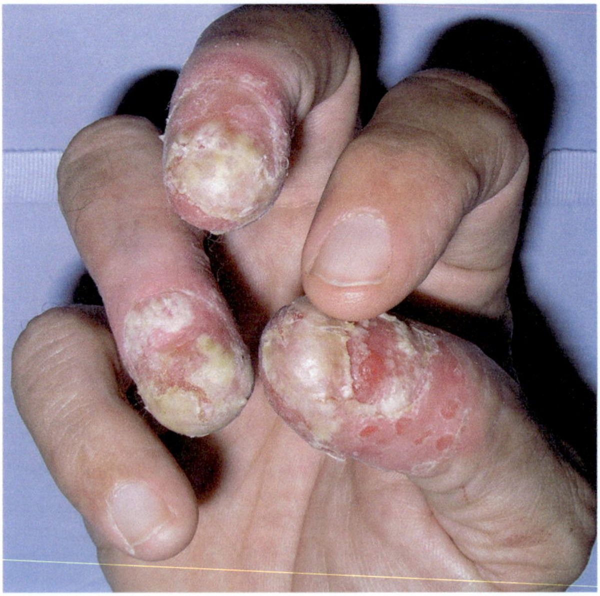

Fig. 14.25 Hallopeau's acrodermatitis continua in a 77-year-old man. Acute inflammation, pustules, and nail plate destruction involving three digits

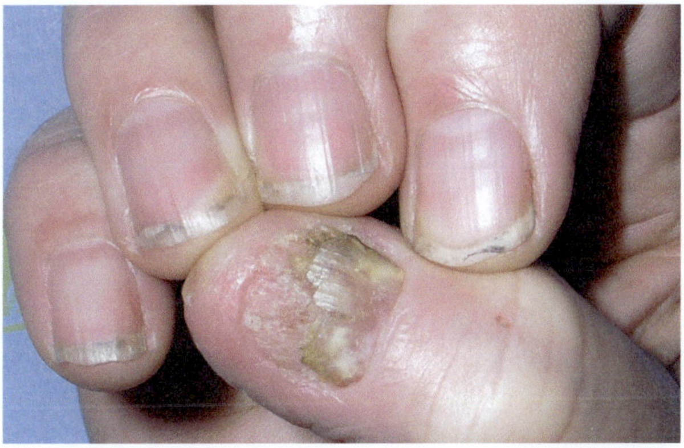

Fig. 14.26 Hallopeau's acrodermatitis continua in a 62-year-old man. The acute episode is remitting and the digit shows mild periungual inflammation with onycholysis and scaling of the nail bed

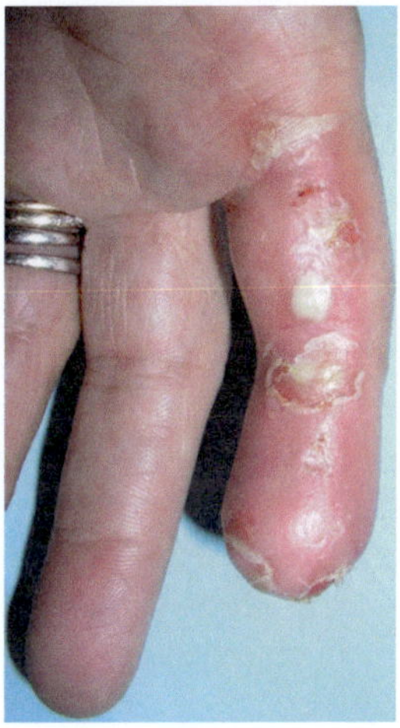

Fig. 14.27 Hallopeau's acrodermatitis continua in a 74-year-old woman. Inflammation and pustules along the digit

- Look at the knees and elbows, as well as at the scalp and folds, in search of signs of psoriasis.
- Look at the plantar skin in order to rule out palmoplantar keratoderma in children and tinea pedis in the elderly.
- Ask for family or personal history of psoriasis.
- Exclude fungal infection by mycology.

Summary for the Clinician

- Do not forget that psoriasis may be limited to the nails both in children and in the elderly.
- Nail symptoms of psoriasis may be unusual in children, with nail thickening as the main sign.

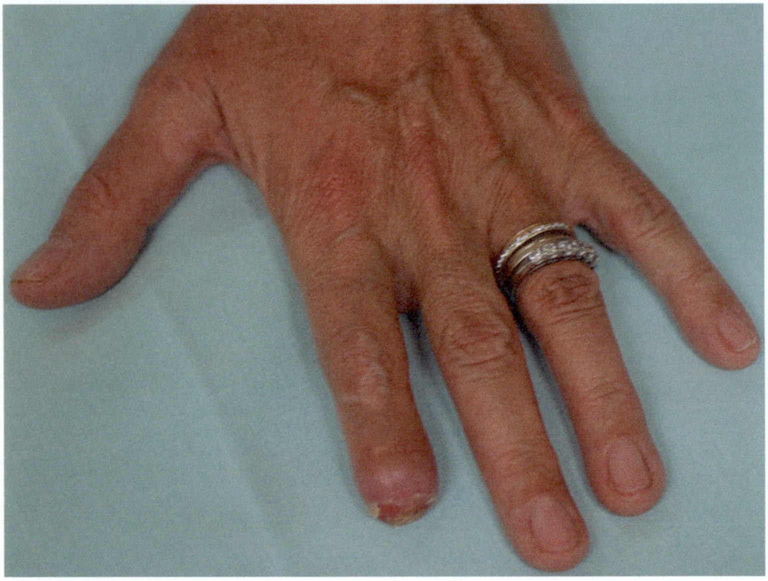

Fig. 14.28 Same patient of Fig. 14.27: frontal view of the hand shows the severe acro-osteolysis with absence of the nail apparatus

- Relapsing pustular inflammation of one digit, with involvement of the periungual skin and nail bed in an adult patient, is suggestive for Hallopeau's acrodermatitis continua.
- The presence of joint pain and swelling of the distal phalanges, which in young and adults with nail psoriasis may be a sign of joint involvement, is not common in elderly, who commonly have sign of arthrosis.

References

1. Kumar B, Jain R, Sandhu K, et al. Epidemiology of childhood psoriasis: a study of 419 patients from northern India. Int J Dermatol. 2004;43:654–8.
2. al-Fouzan AS, Nanda A. A survey of childhood psoriasis in Kuwait. Pediatr Dermatol. 1994;11:116–9.
3. Nanda A, Kaur S, Kaur I, et al. Childhood psoriasis: an epidemiologic survey of 112 patients. Pediatr Dermatol. 1990;7:19–21.
4. Al-Mutairi N, Manchanda Y, Nour-Eldin O. Nail changes in childhood psoriasis: a study from Kuwait. Pediatr Dermatol. 2007;24:7–10.
5. Sehyan M, Coskun BK, Saglam H, et al. Psoriasis in childhood and adolescence: evaluation of demographic and clinical features. Pediatr Int. 2006;48:525–30.
6. Wu Y, Liu H-J, Huang C-Z, et al. Childhood psoriasis: a study of 137 cases from central China. World J Pediatr. 2010;6:260–4.
7. de Chiam LYT, de Jager MEA, Giam YC. Juvenile psoriasis in European and Asian children: similarities and differences. Br J Dermatol. 2011;164:1101–3.
8. Mercy K, Kwasny M, Cordoro KM, et al. Clinical manifestations of pediatric psoriasis: results of a multicenter study in the United States. Pediatr Dermatol. 2013;30:424–8.

9. Kwon HH, Kwon IH, Youn JI. Clinical study of psoriasis occurring over the age of 60 years: is elderly-onset psoriasis a distinct subtype? Int J Dermatol. 2012;51:53–8.
10. Piraccini BM, Tosti A, Iorizzo M, Misciali C. Pustular psoriasis of the nails: treatment and long term follow-up of 46 patients. Br J Dermatol. 2001;144:1000–5.
11. Piraccini BM, Starace M, Bruni F. Onychomycosis in children. Exp Rev Dermatol. 2012;7:569–78.
12. Iorizzo M, Vincenzi C, Smith FJ, Wilson NJ, Tosti A. Pachyonychia congenita type I presenting with subtle nail changes. Pediatr Dermatol. 2009;26:492–3.
13. Tosti A, Peluso AM, Zucchelli V. Clinical features and long-term follow-up of 20 cases of parakeratosis pustulosa. Pediatr Dermatol. 1998;15:259–63.
14. Gordon KA, Vega JM, Tosti A. Trachyonychia: a comprehensive review. Indian J Dermatol Venereol Leprol. 2011;77:640–5.
15. Piraccini BM, Bruni F, Starace M. Dermoscopy of non-skin cancer nail disorders. Dermatol Ther. 2012;25:594–602.
16. Piraccini BM, Balestri R, Starace M, Rech G. Nail digital dermoscopy (onychoscopy) in the diagnosis of onychomycosis. J Eur Acad Dermatol Venereol. 2013;27:509–13.
17. Combemale P, Baran R, Fléchaire A, Boutet B. Psoriatic acro-osteolysis. Exclusive subungual pustular form associated with distant psoriasis vulgaris. Ann Dermatol Venereol. 1989;116:555–8.

How to Choose My Treatment

15

Anna Quinn Hare, Julie Jefferson, and Phoebe Rich

Contents

Key Features

- Selecting an optimal treatment for patients with nail psoriasis is as much art as science.
- Choice of nail psoriasis treatment depends on many factors which are either patient related or psoriasis disease related.
- The extent and severity of nail psoriasis and the impact on quality of life are important in choosing a therapy for nail psoriasis.

Selecting an optimal treatment for patients with nail psoriasis is as much art as science. We present a rational stepwise approach for choosing nail psoriasis therapy by focusing on patient characteristics and nail features and severity and highlighting

A.Q. Hare, MD • P. Rich, MD (✉)
Department of Dermatology, Oregon Health and Science University, Portland, OR, USA
e-mail: anna.hare@gmail.com; phoeberich@aol.com, allie@phoeberichmd.com

J. Jefferson, MD
Department of Dermatology, Johns Hopkins Medicine, Baltimore, MD, USA
e-mail: jjeffe16@jhmi.edu

D. Rigopoulos, A. Tosti (eds.), *Nail Psoriasis: From A to Z*,
DOI 10.1007/978-3-319-08810-5_15

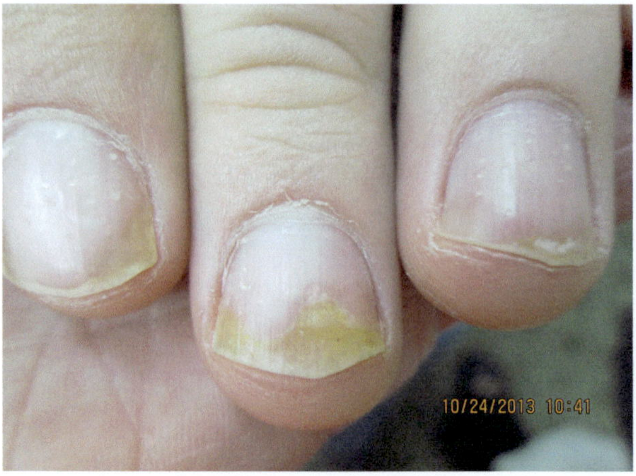

Fig. 15.1 Nail matrix psoriasis, features of pitting (depressions in the nail plate), and psoriatic leukonychia (smooth white spots in the nail plate)

current and emerging treatments for nail psoriasis. While there are currently no treatments that are FDA approved specifically for the treatment of psoriatic nails, the literature is replete with studies of various treatments. Many excellent comprehensive reviews of clinical trials evaluating efficacy of topical and systemic drugs used to treat nail psoriasis have been published, and a PubMed search resulted in over 3,000 studies that look at some aspect of nail psoriasis treatment and it is not our intention to review all of those studies [1–5].

Nail psoriasis, which affects 80–90 % of psoriatics at some time during their life, can be a frustration and a challenge for patient and physician alike [6, 7]. Psoriasis affects the nails in 10–50 % of psoriatics and occasionally nail psoriasis can be the sole feature or the presenting clinical finding of cutaneous psoriasis. A recent large study of pediatric patients found a 39 % prevalence of nail psoriasis [8]. Nail psoriasis severity is positively correlated with duration, extent and severity of plaque psoriasis, and with psoriatic arthritis (PsA) [9]. In fact, studies show a 70 % prevalence of nail PsO in patients with PsA, and in some cases the nail involvement occurs early in the disease process and may be predictive of subsequent PsA development [10, 11].

Healthy nails are important for protecting the digits, assisting in tasks that require dexterity, and making the hands more efficient as tools. Psoriatic nail dystrophy can negatively affect occupational activities and hobbies. Moreover, unsightly fingernail psoriasis can cause psychological distress and may cause patients to avoid certain activities and social situations [12]. Thus, nail psoriasis impairs nail function and appearance and is a burden for patients by seriously impacting quality of life as it interferes with occupational, social, and recreational activities [13, 14].

As with other nail disorders, the clinical appearance of the nail depends on which part of the nail unit is involved with psoriatic inflammation. Psoriatic inflammation can involve the nail bed, nail matrix, and nail fold, resulting in different clinical findings accordingly. Nail bed psoriasis is characterized by onycholysis and associated features of oil drop/salmon patch dyschromia, splinter hemorrhages, and nail bed hyperkeratosis (Figs. 15.1 and 15.2). The hallmark of nail matrix psoriasis is pitting and associated features of crumbling and psoriatic leukonychia which are the same process involving different portions of the matrix and for different durations. Both nail bed and nail matrix psoriasis present the challenge of local delivery of drug to the part of the nail unit responsible for the nail changes. For that reason, the

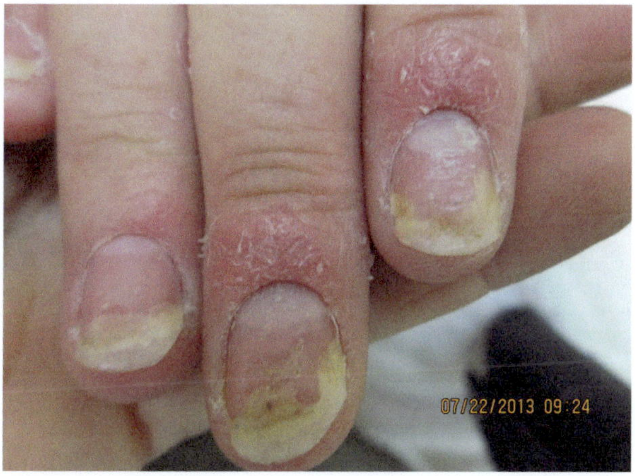

Fig. 15.2 Nail bed psoriasis, features of onycholysis, and oil drop discoloration

nail bed and nail matrix may respond differently to some nail psoriasis treatments. Psoriasis of the proximal and lateral nail folds can result in cuticle loss and lead to psoriatic paronychia. When nail fold attachment to nail plate is altered by psoriasis involving the nail folds, irregularities of the surface of the nail plate is seen as similar to other types of chronic paronychia.

The diagnosis of nail psoriasis is generally not difficult for an experienced dermatologist, especially in the setting of plaque psoriasis. The most common and most important mimic of nail psoriasis is onychomycosis. To further complicate the matter roughly, one third of patients with nail psoriasis have concomitant nail fungus [15–18].

15.1 Choice of Treatment of Nail Psoriasis

The choice of nail psoriasis treatment depends on many factors which are either patient related or psoriasis disease related. Just as psoriasis in other cutaneous locations such as scalp, genital, and palms present unique challenges to treatment, nails can be difficult to treat due to the anatomic and physiologic properties of the nail unit. There are a few first steps that most of nail psoriasis patients benefit from.

1. Education about the nail psoriasis disease process including nail growth rate and timeline for improvement is important. Patients like to know the landscape of treatment options and the risks, benefits, and limitations of various treatment strategies.
2. Assessment of the extent of nail disease and the impact it has on their occupational and social life quality is an important factor. Some patients are not bothered by even severe nail involvement, whereas others may be significantly impacted by minimal pitting or onycholysis. A patient questionnaire is useful in obtaining this information from the patient (Fig. 15.3).
3. Basic nail care is essential for all nail psoriasis patients. Over manipulation can koebnerize the psoriasis and impede progress. Patients should be instructed to treat their nails gently, wear gloves for wet work and chores, and limit contact with harsh chemical and cosmetic processes.

Nail Psoriasis History Sheet

Please help us be thorough in the treatment of your nail psoriasis by answering the following questions:

Name: ___________________________ Age: _____ Sex: M or F Date: ________

Have you ever been diagnosed with nail psoriasis by a physician? YES ____ NO ____

If yes, what was your approximate date of diagnosis? _________

Locations of current of nail psoriasis:

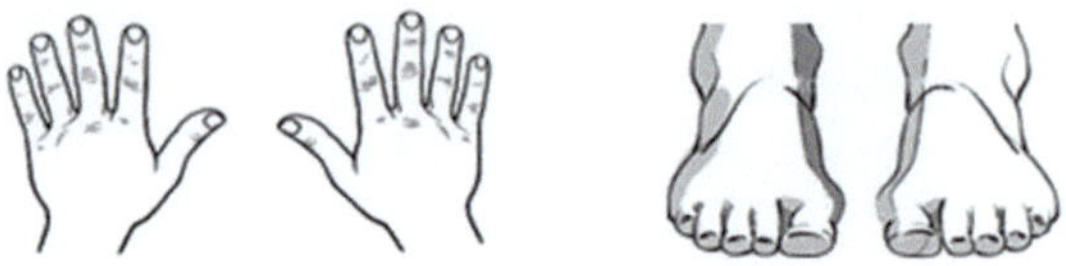

In which other body areas do you have psoriasis (circle all that apply): hands, feet, face, scalp, trunk, arms, legs, genitals

How do you rate severity of your nail psoriasis? (Mark x on line below between 0 and 100)

None 0____100 The worst it could be

What are your nail psoriasis symptoms? (i.e. pain)? ____

How many fingernails are involved? ____ Do you have nail lifting (onycholysis)? ____ Do you have nail depressions (pits)? ____

Do you have joint pain? YES _____ NO_____ If yes, where do you have the joint pain? ___________

Does your body feel stiff when you wake up? YES _____ NO _____

Have you ever been diagnosed with psoriatic arthritis? YES _____ NO _____

Does your nail psoriasis affect your job or personal life? YES _____ NO ____ Please circle all that apply: Trouble doing your job, Problems at school, social activities like dating, family activities, intimate contact, sport activities: swimming, running, biking, choice of vacation, other ___________

Previous treatments: please circle all you have tried:

Local treatment: Topical cortisone, Tazorac, Protopic, calcipotriene (Dovinex), tar, intralesional cortisone (shots around nail) UV light, Laser, other light based treatment, other topicals.

Systemic medications: Methotrexate, Acetretin (previously Soriatane) cyclosporine.

Biologics: Enbrel, Humira, Remicade, Stelara, biologics in a clinical trial

Which of the above treatments were helpful? ____

Did you have side effects with any of the medications used to treat your psoriasis?

What treatment are you currently using for your psoriasis/psoriatic arthritis? Please include frequency and duration of treatments.

Fig. 15.3 Nail psoriasis questionnaire

Treatment of nail psoriasis can be divided into topical therapy, intralesional therapy, devices, and systemic (traditional and biologic) therapy. Rather than repeat the long lists of studies and data presented in other extensive review articles, these categories of nail psoriasis therapy will be summarized. There are currently no drugs approved by the FDA specifically for the indication of nail psoriasis.

15.1.1 Topical Therapy for Nail Psoriasis

Patients who are minimally bothered by their nail psoriasis and who have had no previous therapy for their nails should be given a trial of topical therapy as first line. Many different topical treatments have been used to treat nail psoriasis in the form of solutions, creams, ointments, lacquers, gels, and foams, both with and without occlusion. The most well-studied drugs for topical treatment of nail psoriasis are clobetasol solution and lacquer [19], tazarotene [20, 21], and calcipotriol (Vitamin D3) [22]. Additional small studies have been published on tacrolimus, dithranol [23], topical fluorouracil [24], and cyclosporine [25]. A recent report showed efficacy of indigo naturalis in improving nail psoriasis in children [26].

15.1.2 Intralesional Therapy for Nail Psoriasis

For patients who have mild to moderate nail psoriasis not responding to topical therapy, intralesional cortisone is appropriate. Intralesional injections of low-dose corticosteroid are considered by some to be the mainstay of local treatment of nail psoriasis. Typically, triamcinolone at doses from 2.5 to 10 mg/cc is injected slowly with a 30 gauge needle into the proximal and lateral nail folds every 4–8 weeks [15]. It is not a painful procedure when performed carefully. It helps to cool the skin prior to the injections and to inject superficially into the nail folds so the drug can diffuse to the matrix and nail bed. Direct injection into the nail matrix or nail bed is painful, causes subungual hemorrhages, and is not necessary for successful therapy.

15.1.3 Devices for Nail Psoriasis Therapy

When light-based therapy (UVA, UVB, and PUVA) is used to clear plaque psoriasis, the nails will often improve over time, but there is very little data on nails alone [27]. Superficial X-ray and Grenz Ray have been used historically and shown to be effective but has since fallen out of favor [28]. More recently, 595 pulse dye laser (PDL) has shown efficacy in some small studies [29, 30]. Photodynamic therapy (PDT) using methyl-aminolevulinic acid with PDL 595 did not add any benefit over PDL alone [31].

15.1.4 Systemic Treatment of Nail Psoriasis

Patients with severe nail psoriasis who have not responded to local therapy or who have widespread plaque psoriasis and/or PsA will usually benefit from systemic therapy with either traditional agents such as methotrexate or with biologics. Acitretin, an oral retinoid, has been shown to benefit nail psoriasis at very low dose 0.2–0.3 mg/kg/day [32] and also at 0.5 mg/kg when used with urea nail lacquer [33]. Although methotrexate and cyclosporine have been shown to be effective in psoriasis vulgaris, there are very few trials that look at nail psoriasis [34–37].

15.1.5 Biologics

The past decade has ushered in the era of biologics, which are highly effective and safe in the treatment of psoriasis and psoriatic arthritis. There is data that infliximab [38], adalimumab [39], etanercept [40, 41], golumumab [42], alefacept [43], and ustekinumab [44] all show significant efficacy in improving nail psoriasis.

While the extent and severity of nail psoriasis and the impact on quality of life are important in choosing a therapy for nail psoriasis, other factors should also be considered. Obviously the efficacy and safety of a particular therapy for nail

Table 15.1 Factors that guide and determine nail psoriasis treatments

Important factors in the choice of treatment for nail psoriasis
Age of patient
Previously used treatments
Sex, pregnancy, or nursing
Medical history/medications/comorbidity, TB risk, infection risk, contraindications
Severity of nail disease based on symptoms such as pain
Impact on quality of life caused by the nail disease
Psychological factors impact on quality of life
Extent of skin disease (BSA, PASI, NAPPA)
Presence of psoriatic arthritis (PsA)
Cost of therapy
Convenience of treatment
Motivation of patient
Availability of treatment
Resources available to pay for therapy
Risk vs. benefit for each patient

psoriasis is important, as are patient acceptance, ease of administration, convenience, and cost, which are also considerations when selecting a treatment for nail psoriasis (Table 15.1).

References

1. Reich K. Approach to managing patients with nail psoriasis. J Eur Acad Dermatol Venereol. 2009;23:15–21.
2. de Vries AC, Bogaards NA, Hooft L, Velema M, Pasch M, Lebwohl M, Spuls PI. Interventions for nail psoriasis. Cochrane Database Syst Rev. 2013;(1):CD007633.
3. Tan ES, Chong WS, Tey HL. Nail psoriasis: a review. Am J Clin Dermatol. 2012;13(6):375–88.
4. Oram Y, Akkaya AD. Treatment of nail psoriasis: common concepts and new trends. Dermatol Res Pract. 2013;2013:1–13.
5. Demirsoy EO, Kıran R, Salman S, et al. Effectiveness of systemic treatment agents on psoriatic nails: a comparative study. J Drugs Dermatol. 2013;12(9):1039–43.
6. Jiaravuthisan MM, Dasseville D, Vender RB, et al. Psoriasis of the nail: anatomy, pathology, clinical presentation, and a review of the literature on therapy. J Am Acad Dermatol. 2007;57:1–27.
7. Augustin M, Krüger K, Radtke MA, Schwippl I, Reich K. Disease severity, quality of life and health care in plaque-type psoriasis: a multicenter cross-sectional study in Germany. Dermatology. 2008;216(4):366–72.
8. Mercy M, Kwasny M, Cordoro KM, et al. Clinical manifestations of pediatric psoriasis: results of a multicenter study in the United States. Pediatr Dermatol. 2013;30(4):424–8.
9. Hallaji Z, Babaeijandaghi F, Akbarzadeh M, et al. A significant association exists between the severity of nail and skin involvement in psoriasis. J Am Acad Dermatol. 2012;66:e12–3.
10. Van den Bosch F, Manger B, Goupille P, et al. Effectiveness of adalimumab in treating patients with active psoriatic arthritis and predictors of good clinical responses for arthritis, skin and nail lesions. Ann Rheum Dis. 2010;69:394–9.
11. Maejima H, Taniguchi T, Watarai A, Katsuoka K. Evaluation of nail disease in psoriatic arthritis by using a modified nail psoriasis severity score index. Int J Dermatol. 2010;49(8):901–6.

12. de Jong EM, Seegers BA, Gulinck MK, et al. Psoriasis of the nails associated with disability in a large number of patients: results of a recent interview with 1,728 patients. Dermatology. 1996;193:300–3.
13. Augustin M, Krüger K, Radtke MA, Schwippl I, Reich K. Disease severity, quality of life and health care in plaquetype psoriasis: a multicenter cross-sectional study in Germany. Dermatology. 2008;216(4):366–72.
14. de Berker D. Management of psoriatic nail disease. Semin Cutan Med Surg. 2009;28(1):39–43.
15. Gupta AK, Lynde CW, Jain HC, et al. A higher prevalence of onychomycosis in psoriatics compared with non-psoriatics: a multicenter study. Br J Dermatol. 1997;136:786–9.
16. Sánchez-Regaña M, Videla S, Villoria J, et al. Prevalence of fungal involvement in a series of patients with psoriasis. Clin Exp Dermatol. 2008;33:194–5.
17. Sais G, Jucglà A, Peyri J. Prevalence of dermatophyte onychomycosis in Spain: a cross-sectional study. Br J Dermatol. 1995;132:758–61.
18. Vender RB, Lynde CW, Poulin Y. Prevalence and epidemiology of onychomycosis. J Cutan Med Surg. 2006;10:S28–33.
19. Sánchez Regaña M, Martín Ezquerra G, Umbert Millet P, Llambí Mateos F. Treatment of nail psoriasis with 8% clobetasol nail lacquer: positive experience in 10 patients,". J Eur Acad Dermatol Venereol. 2005;19(5):573–7.
20. De Simone C, Maiorino A, Tassone F, D'Agostino M, Caldarola G. Tacrolimus 0.1% ointment in nail psoriasis: a randomized controlled open-label study. J Eur Acad Dermatol Venereol. 2013;27(8):1003–6.
21. Rigopoulos D, Gregoriou S, Katsambas A. Treatment of psoriatic nails with tazarotene cream 0.1 % vs. clobetasol propionate 0.05 % cream: a double-blind study. Acta Derm Venereol. 2007;87(2):167–8.
22. Tosti A, Piraccini BM, Cameli N, et al. Calcipotriol ointment in nail psoriasis: a controlled double-blind comparison with betamethasone dipropionate and salicylic acid. Br J Dermatol. 1998;139(4):655–9.
23. Yamamoto T, Katayama I, Nishioka K. Topical anthralin therapy for refractory nail psoriasis. J Dermatol. 1998;25(4):231–3.
24. Fredriksson T. Topically applied fluorouracil in the treatment of psoriatic nails. Arch Dermatol. 1974;110(5):735–6.
25. Cannavò SP, Guarneri F, Vaccaro M, Borgia F, Guarneri B. Treatment of psoriatic nails with topical cyclosporin: a prospective, randomized placebo-controlled study. Dermatology. 2003;206(2):153–6.
26. Liang CY, Lin TY, Lin YK. Successful treatment of pediatric nail psoriasis with periodic pustular eruption using topical indigo naturalis oil extract. Pediatr Dermatol. 2013;30:117–9.
27. Marx JL, Scher RK. Response of psoriatic nails to oral photochemotherapy. Arch Dermatol. 1980;116(9):1023–4.
28. Rados J, Dobrić I, Pasić A, Lipozencić J, Ledić-Drvar D, Stajminger G. Normalization in the appearance of severely damaged psoriatic nails using soft x-rays. A case report,". Acta Dermatovenerol Croat. 2007;15:27–32.
29. Oram Y, Karincaoğlu Y, Koyuncu E, Kaharaman F. Pulsed dye laser in the treatment of nail psoriasis. Dermatol Surg. 2010;36(3):377–81.
30. Treewittayapoom C, Singvahanont P, Chanprapaph K, Haneke E. The effect of different pulse durations in the treatment of nail psoriasis with 595-nm pulsed dye laser: a randomized, double-blind, intrapatient left-to-right study. J Am Acad Dermatol. 2012;66:807–12.
31. Fernández-Guarino M, Harto A, Sánchez-Ronco M, García-Morales I, Jaén P. Pulsed dye laser vs. photodynamic therapy in the treatment of refractory nail psoriasis: a comparative pilot study. J Eur Acad Dermatol Venereol. 2009;23(8):891–5.
32. Tosti A, Ricotti C, Romanelli P, Cameli N, Piraccini BM. Evaluation of the efficacy of acitretin therapy for nail psoriasis. Arch Dermatol. 2009;145(3):269–71.
33. Ricceri F, Pescitelli L, Tripo L, Bassi A, Prignano F. Treatment of severe nail psoriasis with acitretin: an impressive therapeutic result. Dermatol Ther. 2013;26:77–8.
34. Feliciani C, Zampetti A, Forleo P, et al. Nail psoriasis: combined therapy with systemic cyclosporin and topical calcipotriol. J Cutan Med Surg. 2004;8(2):122–5.

35. Mahrle G, Schulze HJ, Färber L, Weidinger G, Steigleder GK. Low-dose short-term cyclosporine versus etretinate in psoriasis: improvement of skin, nail, and joint involvement. J Am Acad Dermatol. 1995;32:78–88.
36. Sánchez-Regaña M, Sola-Ortigosa J, Alsina-Gibert M, Vidal-Fernández M, Umbert-Millet P. Nail psoriasis: a retrospective study on the effectiveness of systemic treatments (classical and biological therapy). J Eur Acad Dermatol Venereol. 2011;25(5):579–88.
37. Gümüşel M, Özdemir M, Mevlitoğlu I, Bodur S. Evaluation of the efficacy of methotrexate and cyclosporine therapies on psoriatic nails: a one-blind, randomized study. J Eur Acad Dermatol Venereol. 2011;25:1080–4.
38. Rich P, Griffiths CEM, Reich K, et al. Baseline nail disease in patients with moderate to severe psoriasis and response to treatment with infliximab during 1 year. J Am Acad Dermatol. 2008;58(2):224–31.
39. Van den Bosch F, Manger B, Goupille P, et al. Effectiveness of adalimumab in treating patients with active psoriatic arthritis and predictors of good clinical responses for arthritis, skin and nail lesions. Ann Rheum Dis. 2010;69(2):394–9.
40. Ortonne JP, Paul C, Berardesca E, Marino V, Gallo G, Brault Y, Germain JM. A 24-week randomized clinical trial investigating the efficacy and safety of two doses of etanercept in nail psoriasis. Br J Dermatol. 2013;168(5):1080–7.
41. Luger TA, Barker J, Lambert J, et al. Sustained improvement in joint pain and nail symptoms with etanercept therapy in patients with moderate-to-severe psoriasis. J Eur Acad Dermatol Venereol. 2009;23(8):896–904.
42. Kavanaugh A, Mclnnes I, Mease P, et al. Golimumab, a new human tumor necrosis factor α antibody, administered every four weeks as a subcutaneous injection in psoriatic arthritis: twenty-four-week efficacy and safety results of a randomized, placebo-controlled study. Arthritis Rheum. 2009;60(4):976–86.
43. Parrish CA, Sobera JO, Robbins CM, Cantrell WC, Desmond RA, Elewski BE. Alefacept in the treatment of psoriatic nail disease: a proof of concept study. J Drugs Dermatol. 2006;5(4):339–40.
44. Rich P, Bourcier M, Sofen H, Fakharzadeh S, Wasfi Y, Wang Y, Kerkmann U, Ghislain P-D, Poulin Y, The PHOENIX 1 Investigators. Ustekinumab improves nail disease in patients with moderate-to-severe psoriasis: results from PHOENIX 1. Br J Dermatol. 2014;170:398–407.

What Is the Future?

16

Dimitris Rigopoulos and Antonella Tosti

Content

Key Features

- The nail plate acts like a barrier for topical treatment.
- Side effects of systemic treatment are a concern for the patients.
- Interactions of systemic drugs are also a problem for the psoriatic patient.
- New formulations with better penetration, no side effects and no interaction are needed.

The major problem when treating nail psoriasis is either the difficulty of the topical medications to present their therapeutic efficacy or the side effects of the systematically administrated drugs.

Topical medications must penetrate the nail plate which in normal conditions presents unique barrier properties, taking in consideration also that in psoriasis it can be thickened due to the hyperkeratosis of the nail bed, increasing difficulties in acting properly.

D. Rigopoulos, MD (✉)
Department of Dermatology, Athens University School of Medicine, Athens, Greece
e-mail: drigop@hol.gr

A. Tosti, MD
Department of Dermatology and Cutaneous Surgery, University of Miami
Miller School of Medicine, Miami, FL, USA
e-mail: antonella.tosti@unibo.it

D. Rigopoulos, A. Tosti (eds.), *Nail Psoriasis: From A to Z*,
DOI 10.1007/978-3-319-08810-5_16

Systemic drugs have three major problems. The first has to deal with side effects of these drugs, the second with interactions with other systemic medications that these patients are probably receiving, and the third with the lack of on-label indication for nail psoriasis. The latter is a major problem when the patient has isolated nail involvement.

So, major improvement for topical drugs would be solving penetration problems and for systemic ones would be creating new drugs with few or no side effects and no interactions.

Most of the information concerning penetration enhancing of topical medication comes from studies with antifungal drugs, and these vehicles can probably be tested in the future for delivering steroids or other psoriasis-effective drugs.

Ciclopirox dissolved in a lipid diffusion enhancer (utilizing the lipid pathway of the nail) proved to be concentrated in deep nail layers and nail bed in a statistical significant greater concentration than the same drug in the form of a lacquer [1]. Thiourea, which improves the solubility and due to this effect nail penetration, has also been used as an enhancer of ciclopirox olamine through the nail plate [2]. Low-molecular-weight polyethylene glycols, due to their ability to lead to greater water uptake and swelling of the nail, can be used as trans-ungual permeation enhancers either alone or in combination with iontophoresis [3]. Hydrophobins A-C (proteins rich in cysteine) in a concentration of 0.1 % have been studied on cadaver nails, and they proved to enhance the permeability of terbinafine 10 % solution in 60 % ethanol/water [4]. Pretreatment of the nail plate with phosphoric acid 1 or 10 % (w/w) for a short duration (60 s) can be a potential method for improving the efficiency of topical monotherapy treatment for nail disease according to the authors of a study which tried to study the increase of the delivery into and across the human nail plate of terbinafine hydrochloride and 5-fluorouracil [5]. According to the authors of a study published recently which tested the ability of a formulation of triamcinolone (containing *N*-acetylcysteine – as penetration enhancer and Pluronic F-127 – with gelling properties and increase ability of drugs solubility) to deliver the active ingredient across the human nail, aqueous-based nail lacquers represent a superior formulation strategy in human nail delivery [6]. The addition of inorganic salts (0.5 M), due to their ability to augment the hydration of the nail plate and also increase the thermodynamic activity of the drug, enhanced terbinafine absorption three to five times through the nail, while the drug load was increased four up to seven times. Interestingly, increase of the concentration of the inorganic salts to 1 M (but not more) increased the effect [7]. In vitro study on human nail clippings of the enhancing properties of thioglycolic acid and urea hydrogen peroxide revealed that thioglycolic acid but not urea hydrogen peroxide could increase the permeability of caffeine and methylparaben, four- and twofolds, respectively. The mode of action of both enhancers is expressed via the disruption of keratin disulfide bonds and the formation of pores that provide more "open" drug transport channels [8].

Enhancing drug penetration can also be achieved through mechanical modalities like ultrasounds. A slip-in device consisting of an ultrasound transducer and a drug delivery compartment above each toenail was used. The device was connected to a computer and canine nails were used. A stereomicroscope was used to access the quantity of the drug-mimicking compound and was delivered through the nail plate which was increased by this method [9].

What remains to be tested and subsequently proved is the efficacy of the abovementioned chemical enhancers and mechanical modalities with drugs that can be effective with nail psoriasis.

References

1. Haffez F, Hui X, Selner M, et al. Ciclopirox delivery into the human nail plate using novel lipid diffusion enhancers. Drug Dev Ind Pharm. 2013;19:21–32.
2. Palliyi B, Lebo DB, Patel PR. A preformulation strategy for the selection of penetration enhancers for a transungual formulation. AAPS PharmSciTech. 2013;14(2):682–91.
3. Nair AB, Chakraborty B, Murthy SN. Effect of polyethylene glycols on the trans-ungual delivery of terbinafine. Curr Drug Deliv. 2010;7(5):407–14.
4. Vejnovic I, Huonder C, Betz G. Permeation studies of novel Terbinafine formulations containing hydrophobins through human nails in vitro. Int J Pharm. 2010;397(1–2):67–76.
5. Vaka SR, Murthy SN, O'Haver JH, et al. A platform for predicting and enhancing model drug delivery across the human nail plate. Drug Dev Ind Pharm. 2011;37(1):72–9.
6. Nogueiras-Nieto L, Delgado-Charro M, Otero-Espinar FJ. Thermogelling hydrogels of cyclodextrins/poloxamer polypseudorotaxanes as aqueous-based nail lacquers: application to the delivery of triamcinolone acetonide and ciclopirox olamine. Eur J Pharm Biopharm. 2013;83(3):370–7.
7. Nair AB, Sammeta SM, Vaka SR, et al. A study on the effect of inorganic salts in transungual drug delivery of terbinafine. J Pharm Pharmacol. 2009;61(4):431–7.
8. Brown MB, Khengar RH, Turner RB, et al. Overcoming the nail barrier: a systematic investigation of ungula chemical penetration enhancement. Int J Pharm. 2009;370(1–2):61–7.
9. Abadi D, Zderic V. Ultrasound-mediated nail drug delivery system. J Ultrasound Med. 2011;30(12):1723–30.

MIX
Papier aus verantwortungsvollen Quellen
Paper from responsible sources
FSC® C105338
FSC
www.fsc.org

If you have any concerns about our products,
you can contact us on
ProductSafety@springernature.com

In case Publisher is established outside the EU,
the EU authorized representative is:
Springer Nature Customer Service Center GmbH
Europaplatz 3, 69115 Heidelberg, Germany

Printed by Libri Plureos GmbH
in Hamburg, Germany